Praise for *Supermodel YOU*

*Being a father of three young children, I am eternally grateful that
Sarah DeAnna has written such an important and life-affirm*⌐   ⌐*k!
In our present-day Photoshop/outside-in-approach* ⌐⌐*¹*
wellness, and self-esteem, Sarah demystifies, d⌐*ʰ*   ⌐*al
steps to reclaiming our power.* **Super**⌐   ⌐
both wisdom and wit to live ⌐

— **Dr. Darren R. Weissman**,
of The LifeLine Techniqu⌐

Supermodel YOU is a compel⌐   ⌐*ⱶat takes us on a
journey of supermodel transformation! A terrific guide that shares
the keys to unlocking the inner model within all of us.*

— **John Tew,** The Beauté Guru, makeup artist to the stars

*As a celebrity fashion stylist, I know everyone wants that sexy,
svelte model physique.* **Supermodel YOU** *shows you how
it's done in a healthy, happy way.*

— **Marcellas Reynolds,** E! network and CNN correspondent

*As a gorgeous, successful model, Sarah DeAnna is uniquely
qualified to shepherd us along the often-mystifying road to
our "skinniest," healthiest selves. Now that's chic!*

— **Amanda Luttrell Garrigus**, fashion journalist
and *E! News* correspondent

True definition of <u>*sexy*</u> *is someone like Sarah DeAnna who finally brings forth
the* <u>*awareness*</u> *needed for all to be healthy. Whether you are a model trying
to compete in this crazy industry or someone who is searching for how to be
healthy and not sacrifice your life but rather enjoy it . . . this book is for you.
I've shot thousands of young aspiring models for over 20 years and believe in
this book more than words can say, as I have seen so much unnecessary body
abuse. I am so inspired by Sarah DeAnna's compassion and* **Supermodel YOU**
that I will personally <u>*give*</u> *it out to every aspiring model I shoot in the future!*

— **Greg James,** photographer

*Sarah DeAnna's outlook is refreshing, appealing, and a much-needed
perspective in our culture today. Not only is she fierce in her approach, she
combines real-life circumstances that women often face with her own unique
experiences as a supermodel. Above all, Sarah DeAnna delivers a message
that our culture is desperate to hear: You don't have to be a model, or a size 0,
or a huge success on the runway for you to learn to love the skin you are in.*

— **Eric Handler,** co-founder of **www.positivelypositive.com**

After working for years as a celebrity makeup artist and a life coach, I have seen firsthand what it takes to truly be "beautiful" . . . and Sarah DeAnna is it! By ripping apart the supermodel stereotypes and giving us a peek backstage at the fashion show of life, Sarah gives us a real path to rocking our looks! Her Five Keys are a livable, everyday recipe for beauty inside and out.

— **Michelle Phillips,** best-selling author of
The Beauty Blueprint, celebrity makeup artist,
national TV and radio host, and keynote speaker

I am really excited about this book. Why shouldn't health and confidence be easy and fun? I haven't always taken great care of myself, and I've tried the crash-dieting thing, but you can't live your life like that. If I can learn how to look and feel better for life, I can pass that on to my kids.

— **Melissa Lamming**, virtual assistant to the stars,
Assist on the Run LLC

Finally there's someone out there who gives women all over the world the opportunity to learn what it's really like to be a model. Shooting for a magazine is only 10 percent of this glamorous life. The other 90 percent is taking care of yourself so you can be the best of you! I love that **Supermodel YOU** *gives you the Five Keys that will change your life.*

— **Melissa Rose Haro**, *Sports Illustrated*
Rookie of the Year swimsuit model, 2008–2009

I work with and know many models, and above all Sarah DeAnna has the stunning beauty, the mental strength, the intelligence, and—most importantly—the heart of a supermodel. The fashion industry frequently gets blamed for being the root cause of eating disorders. However, models such as Sarah DeAnna who are perfect models of health— physically, mentally, and spiritually—are "super role models" for our society. This is not another redundant health-and-fitness/weight-loss book that encourages fanatic dieting and exercising. In **Supermodel YOU**, *Sarah writes with honestly and love, generously sharing with the world her secrets to achieving one's dream body!*

— **Brenda Vongova**, United Nations Under-Secretary
General for Political Affairs, supermodel trainer,
and founder of the Vongova Bodylift Method

You can be a supermodel. Yes, YOU! It is all about attitude, self-image, and taking care of yourself. **Supermodel YOU** *will show you how to be kind, respectful, and loving to the person who deserves it the most . . . YOU. You only have one body and one mind. Treat yourself right. Treat yourself like a supermodel.*

Author and supermodel Sarah DeAnna is beautiful inside and out. It didn't just happen by itself. Sarah rolled up her sleeves, got busy, and is making an impact on the world. One of the reasons **Supermodel YOU** is inspirational is that Sarah knows of what she speaks. She's been there, done that. Sarah wasn't just handed the life of a supermodel.

Sarah's book will help you bring out the supermodel in YOU. Beauty is a billion-dollar business, and models are the benchmark of beauty. Sure, not every woman can be 5'11" and wear a size 2, but every woman can be the best they can be. This is the message **Supermodel YOU** invokes.

As a filmmaker and former model, I've seen firsthand the casualties of those who didn't take care of themselves. Those were the ones with short-lived careers. When people stereotype fashion models, they think of eating disorders, drug abuse, smokers, spoiled brats, and egg-fragile egos. Sarah debunks this generalization and illustrates that models who have longevity in the beauty business take care of themselves both mentally and physically.

Sarah has discovered Five Keys to channel your inner supermodel. She has given us a valuable gift with **Supermodel YOU.** Don't throw it away. No more excuses. No more low self-esteem. It's time to be proactive. It's time for YOU to actually take charge of your life and not just talk about it. It time to own your beauty and nourish it. It's time for YOU to be beautiful, sexy, smart, and happy. It's time for YOU to become your own supermodel. Yes . . . YOU!

— **Brent Huff,** director of *Chasing Beauty*

I've spent the last 25 years surrounded by tall, skinny, pretty people, some very healthy, some not. Thank God for Sarah DeAnna, a beautiful soul that has taken the time to write a book about how to do it right!

— **Crista Klayman,** agent, L.A. Models,
known for discovering Tyra Banks

As a beauty expert, I feel that true beauty starts from the inside and finds its way out. **Supermodel YOU** *uniquely guides you to get into the sexiest and healthiest shape of your life with results that are long lasting, both from the inside and out.*

— **Roxy,** celebrity and fashion makeup artist

I'm known for helping both people and organizations get the results they want in order to succeed, and I believe Sarah DeAnna's book, **Supermodel YOU,** *can help you get the results you're looking for when it comes to looking and feeling your best.*

— **Tony Jeary,** The RESULTS Guy™

Sarah DeAnna has inspired so many people, including myself, to be the best they can be. And now she inspires YOU with her brilliantly easy steps to becoming the healthier, happier person you deserve to be.

— **Rob Meadows,** Originate CEO and founder;
technology entrepreneur and investor

Sarah DeAnna is the nicest model I've worked with in the business. In addition to being smart and beautiful, she is in incredible shape, with the hair and skin to match. Her book is a must-read for all of us who want to look and feel our best.

— **Trinette Faint**, model, author, and featured Beauty
and Travel blogger for *Harper's Bazaar* and *Marie Claire*

*I believe that looking good is about feeling good, too. And I believe that Sarah DeAnna's book, **Supermodel YOU**, will teach you a thing or two about how to achieve that healthy, happy balance.*

— **Greg Alterman**, Alternative Apparel
founder/Chief Creative Officer

***Supermodel YOU** is about being the super version of yourself, your best, healthiest, and most beautiful self. This book will teach you how to become that supermodel version of YOU, because there's no point in trying to be anybody else.*

— **Julia Lescova**, supermodel, Guess? Girl,
and Model of the World winner

***Supermodel YOU** is a book about women being able to gain full control over their own destiny. In a clear, simple, and engaging style, Sarah DeAnna lays the foundation of how to attain what we social scientists call self-regulation, self-control, or self-actualization. These concepts do not imply "control of the self," for instance, as if the self was "out of control"; rather, they designate the processes human beings recruit when they exert free will in order to become all that they can be.*

Sarah's inspiring message is that all women can become their ideal inner and outer selves by following five key principles that include stress management, varied physical activities, and intelligent eating. She posits that the prerequisite—the very first key principle—for any positive change to occur is self-awareness. Indeed, how can one seek self-improvement if one is oblivious to what needs improvement to start with?

Self-awareness precisely represents my main research area. I am very impressed by Sarah's articulate view of the self-awareness process, which I find to be totally consistent with our current scientific knowledge. Giants in psychology have extensively written on self-awareness and self-control—Albert Bandura and Roy Baumeister come to mind. They, too, suggest that a constant and careful monitoring of the self constitutes the first step in self-change, and this idea has received objective support from numerous scientific studies.

In my view, only Sarah DeAnna could have written this enlightening book dedicated to giving women more power to themselves. First, she is a high-fashion model! Sarah thus provides the reader with tons of colorful examples of how real models successfully set, attain, and maintain personal and professional goals. Second, Sarah possesses this intuitive knowledge of how self-awareness represents the key process that allows models to orchestrate all aspects of their lives (such as eating and exercising) in the most efficient way possible. This key process actually applies to all women and human beings, not just models; Sarah makes this point amply clear, and it most certainly represents the main—very positive—message of her book.

Sarah DeAnna's goal is to empower women not to become mindless beauties but self-intelligent creators of their own lives.

— **Alain Morin, Ph.D.**, Associate Professor, Department of Psychology, Mount Royal University, Calgary, Alberta, Canada

Sarah DeAnna's story will touch your heart! It will inspire you and motivate you toward the joy of taking better care of yourself. This book is a toolbox for the well-being of the best model of you!

— **Agapi Stassinopoulos**, best-selling author of *Unbinding the Heart*

Gandhi once said, "Strength does not come from physical capacity. It comes from an indomitable will." This quote perfectly describes the young girl from Oregon who once sat in my office and told me she would like to be somebody, and help other people realize they were somebody, too. Inward acheivements change outer reality. You go, girl!

— **Nicole Bordeaux**, founder/owner of PhotoGenics Media

Sarah DeAnna's book is a compassionate and deeply personal guide to waking the spirit within the body. It seeks to engage the "five essential intelligences"—physical, mental, emotional, moral, and spiritual. It provides powerful yet simple ways to fully engage each level and pay attention to our bodies' unique patterns, achieving the benefits of expressing our full potential. Sarah demonstrates that when we wake up fully in our bodies and harmonize all five layers, we discover a result that is more than the sum of the parts: we fall deeply in love with being alive and fully present. This book is a warm, funny, encouraging, compassionate, and deeply personal guide to waking every fiber of your body and being.

— **Guru Mirumi, Ph.D.**, member of the Association for Psychological Science

***Supermodel YOU** is your guide to feeling better, looking better, and being your best "supermodel" self. Sarah DeAnna takes us inside the modeling world and teaches us how to eat like, walk like, and think like a supermodel. With humor, straight talk, and illuminating examples, Sarah lets us in on the secrets the supermodels know. I loved **Supermodel YOU**. If you want to be your best self, reading this book will be time well spent.*

— **Irene Rubaum-Keller, LMFT**, author of *Foodaholic*

***Supermodel YOU** is more than a guide to being a supermodel. It's an owners' manual to the body, mind, and spirit.*

— **Ryan Blair**, *New York Times* best-selling author of *Nothing to Lose, Everything to Gain*

SUPERMODEL
YOU

Hay House Titles of Related Interest

SUPERMODEL
YOU

Shockingly Healthy Insider Tips to Bring Out **Your Inner Supermodel**

Sarah DeAnna
with Eve Adamson

HAY HOUSE, INC.
Carlsbad, California • New York City
London • Sydney • Johannesburg
Vancouver • Hong Kong • New Delhi

Published and distributed in the United States by: Hay House, Inc.: www .hayhouse.com® • *Published and distributed in Australia by:* Hay House Australia Pty. Ltd.: www.hayhouse.com.au • *Published and distributed in the United Kingdom by:* Hay House UK, Ltd.: www.hayhouse.co.uk • *Published and distributed in the Republic of South Africa by:* Hay House SA (Pty), Ltd.: www.hayhouse .co.za • *Distributed in Canada by:* Raincoast: www.raincoast.com • *Published in India by:* Hay House Publishers India: www.hayhouse.co.in

Cover design: Patricia Martin-Owen • *Interior design:* Riann Bender
Illustration on page 201: Monika Rofler • *Photo on page 267:* Melissa Rodwell Photography

Library of Congress Cataloging-in-Publication Data

DeAnna, Sarah
  Supermodel you : shockingly healthy insider tips to bring out your inner supermodel / Sarah DeAnna with Eve Adamson. -- 1st ed.
     p. cm.
  ISBN 978-1-4019-4020-1 (tradepaper : alk. paper) -- ISBN 978-1-4019-4021-8 (ebk)
1. Body image in women. 2. Beauty, Personal. 3. Self-consciousness (Awareness)
4. Self-esteem in women. I. Adamson, Eve. II. Title.
  BF697.5.B63D43 2013
  646.70082--dc23

                                   2012042024

Tradepaper ISBN: 978-1-4019-4020-1
Digital ISBN: 978-1-4019-4021-8

16 15 14 13   5 4 3 2
1st edition, April 2013
2nd edition, April 2013

Printed in the United States of America

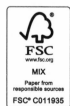

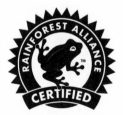

For every woman or girl who has ever dreamed about being a supermodel, or who just wants to have the body, beauty, and attitude of a supermodel.
This book is for YOU!

CONTENTS

PREFACE

Do you ever wonder what it would be like to be a supermodel? To feel incredible and beautiful and sexy and empowered? Maybe you've even daydreamed about the luxurious, glamorous life a supermodel must live. What would it be like? And why can't that be *you?*

Maybe you were one of those little girls who dreamed about being a supermodel someday. Or who looked in the mirror on a confident day and thought: *I'm beautiful! I should be a model!* A lot of little girls dream about this, and most of them go on to have other kinds of careers than modeling. But that doesn't mean you have to let that little-girl dream die.

You are fabulous enough, beautiful enough, *super* enough to be the supermodel version of you. That's what *Supermodel YOU* is all about! All you need to know is what real models do to stay so gorgeous. You don't have to settle for a body, a look, or a life that doesn't feel right to you or that doesn't feel like the best you can possibly be. All you need to know are a few key secrets.

Models don't have it all, of course. We have our issues, our problems, our fat days, our bad-hair days—all of that. But what we do know is how to look good, how to maintain our ideal body weight, and how to rock a room when we walk into it. We have to know these things. It's our profession. We get paid to master this stuff, and despite what you might have heard, many models have shockingly healthy habits that maximize their slammin' bodies, iconic faces, and confident attitudes.

Our tricks and habits are such guarded secrets that a lot of models don't even realize why they work! But I do. I've made it my business to look closely at what I do and to research and grill all my model friends to figure out what *they* do. After tons of reading and watching and questioning, I discovered that there are Five Keys to channeling your inner supermodel. I determined exactly what models do that other people don't necessarily do—how we eat, how we move, how we deal with stress, how we sleep, how we act, even how we think. And now, I'm going to share those secrets with you.

In *Supermodel YOU,* you will learn what the Five Keys are, and how to make them work in your life. You'll also learn how models stay healthy enough to live on the road and still look gorgeous. You'll get supermodel playlists to help you bop through every key, model meal plans so you can see what real models eat, model "exercise" tips (including the fact that most models don't actually exercise), and more. You'll learn what models wear, how they shop, how they snack, and how they pack when they find out at 6 P.M. that they have to fly to Bangkok at 6 A.M. the next day—and how every single one of those things contributes to a supermodel body and a supermodel attitude.

Then you will learn how you can apply those model secrets to your own life. You'll learn how to be *skealthy* (my word for skinny-but-also-healthy), and you'll learn how to walk into a room with *modeltude* (the attitude that models have, knowing they are hot!). With the Five Keys to channeling your inner supermodel, you'll maximize your best possible self. Life will get easier, more glamorous, sexier, and more fun.

Not everyone can be a supermodel by profession. We need doctors, teachers, journalists, scientists . . . and we need YOU. But just because you're still in school or you're a stay-at-home mom or you work in an office doesn't mean you don't deserve to look and feel like a supermodel.

Supermodel YOU is not about looking like me, Cindy Crawford, Gisele Bündchen, a Victoria's Secret Angel, or any other supermodel or girl in a magazine or on TV. Trying to be or look like someone else is just a waste of being *you!* Movie-star legend Judy Garland famously said, "Be a first-rate version of yourself, not a second-rate version of someone else." Scientifically and genetically speaking, there will never be another you, so why not be the most beautiful, sexiest, healthiest, most confident version of yourself possible? This book is about feeling empowered to find yourself and then maximize this, because you own yourself, and only you know how far you can go with your own power.

So drop the self-loathing and low self-esteem. Forget about diets and crazy exercise regimens. All you need are the Five Keys, which are based in science and vetted by models all over the world. The keys are proven, but making them part of your life is fun. You'll get into the model psyche and learn how to adopt the attitude that you are the supermodel version of yourself: beautiful, flawless, fun, sexy, and amazing. You're about to look it, feel it, live it. You're about to achieve Supermodel YOU! Get ready to walk the runway of your life.

■ ■ ■

INTRODUCTION

*No one sees life through your eyes, hears
with your ears, smells through your nose,
tastes with your mouth, feels through your skin,
or is aware of your intuition as acutely as you are.*

— DR. DARREN WEISSMAN, SUPER–HOLISTIC PHYSICIAN AND AUTHOR

I'm Sarah DeAnna, or "Chubbs," as my sisters used to call me! Today, I'm an international fashion model who has walked hundreds of runways and appeared in *Vogue, Elle,* and *Marie Claire,* as well as in many other top fashion magazines. I'm not a doctor, a dietitian, a nutritionist, or a personal trainer. However, I know a lot about what models do to stay thin and beautiful, and that's what I want to share with you in this book.

I also want to dispel some myths. People tend to think models are genetically privileged, born beautiful, naturally skinny . . . in other words, that they aren't like "normal" people and must come from some magical place where everyone is perfect—from Planet Model. I'm here to tell you how untrue this is. But what do I know? Being skinny is all in my (designer) genes, right?

Actually, I am from a teeny-tiny farm town in the Willamette Valley called Jefferson, Oregon. Population: 2,000. The welcome sign as you enter reads: MINT CAPITAL OF THE WORLD. Yes, we grow mint! As if mint doesn't grow wild everywhere. But in Jefferson,

Oregon, we've made it our claim to fame. I was actually the Junior Mint Princess one year at our annual Mint Festival, where we jumped bullfrogs while our parents got drunk on mint-flavored concoctions at the beer garden. Junior Mint Princess wasn't even a title that really existed—my mom was on the committee, so she made it up and then bestowed it on me. There was no vote—believe me, if there had been, one of the popular girls would have been elected. Certainly not me, the little girl from the wrong side of the tracks who grew up catching polliwogs with her sister in the creek next to our house. Back then, I'd certainly never heard of Giorgio Armani, Dolce & Gabbana, or Louis Vuitton. I'd never even seen a Porsche before I moved to California. Maybe it sounds idyllic, like the perfect little small-town existence, but I was far from being anything like a real princess, kissing toads and living in a mint green palace.

When I was in first grade, my siblings and I were taken to a foster home, and my dad was taken to prison. My mother got us back, but she might have been better off without us because of all the responsibilities that suddenly came crashing down. In one day, she went from happy housewife to single mother of four, and this was so hard on her that it broke her. My dad was in and out of prison throughout most of my childhood, and my mom turned to alcohol to pacify her sorrows. I'll never forget that night: she'd gotten two DUIs in less than 24 hours, and when they locked her up, there we were, four little kids waiting at home with both our parents in jail, and nobody came. We were left totally alone.

After my dad went to prison and my mom was dealing with her own grief and anguish most of the time, we had to fend for ourselves, taking care of each other as best we could. We always had a roof over our heads and food, but it certainly wasn't an ideal childhood. (I don't blame my mother. I know she did the best she could in the situation.) We went on welfare and were given food stamps, but to us, "food" meant Twinkies, Ding-Dongs, candy, hot dogs, corn dogs, frozen pizza, Hamburger Helper, soda, Kool-Aid . . . it was basically all packaged, processed stuff kids could make for themselves, but it was also all basically sugar. It wasn't a nutritionally sound diet, but at least we survived.

I grew up eating crap, and feeling like crap, too. I had a lot of stomachaches, and I think I've had about a hundred cavities. I've had bridges, root canals, and fillings galore! My family always said our bad teeth were genetic, but I have a feeling it had something to do with my favorite snack growing up: white bread with half a stick of butter and half a cup of cinnamon-sugar. It was my favorite food ever, but I can't even imagine eating that now! And water? I never drank water! I downed Pepsi, Mountain Dew, Dr. Pepper, Orange Crush, root beer, and Kool-Aid. I loved Kool-Aid! Or rather, I loved the ten cups of sugar I added to the tiny packet of powder!

I'm sure consuming all of this sugar didn't help our behavior. Because my siblings and I didn't really have any discipline or a strong authority figure to help guide us, we became four hell-raisers: the children you didn't want your kids to play with! Aside from smoking cigarettes around age 12 in a failed attempt to look cool, and trying marijuana and alcohol, I managed to avoid going too far down the road that my siblings traveled. At some point, I realized that this wasn't the way to make something of myself. I guess you could say I listened to my gut, and it told me I wanted a better future than what I saw before me. Although I didn't yet know where I was headed, I knew my family's route was never going to get me on the cover of *Vogue* magazine. I knew it wasn't going to get me anywhere I really wanted to go, including out of Jefferson.

I was never good at being bad anyway, so I became a goody-two-shoes overachiever instead. I went from skipping half of one semester of my freshman year to graduating with honors, making me the first and only kid in my family to even finish high school.

MODEL **TALK**

It takes but one positive thought when given a chance to survive and thrive to overpower an entire army of negative thoughts.

— Robert H. Schuller, super–motivational speaker and superpastor

Even though I had already risen well above everyone's expectations—like graduating from high school and from college with an international business marketing and Spanish double major—I was still hungry to do more. I moved to Los Angeles as a UCLA Anderson School of Management hopeful. I don't know if it was because I was tall and strange-looking or if people could sense that I secretly wanted to be a supermodel, but I was often approached by individuals claiming to be model scouts, photographers, and agents. Naturally, I was flattered—who wouldn't be? I wanted to believe I had potential, and I loved that they thought I was beautiful. The $10,000-a-day salary I was promised sounded amazing, but also sounded too good to be true. I was suspicious, and modeling was not my goal, so I blew off all overtures.

Finally, at Starbucks on Melrose Avenue in Hollywood, I met a photographer named James O'Hara, the man I credit for "discovering" me. For some reason I trusted him. Within a few days, James did my first real photo shoot, and then took me to one of Los Angeles's finest modeling agencies. They signed me immediately. I was still very unsure of my ability to model, but underneath all of that insecurity was a little girl who used to dream of being a famous supermodel. But that little-girl dream wasn't really what drove me to accept their offer. It was that I wanted to *be* somebody. I wanted the ability and the voice to make a difference and to help people in need. I wanted to matter! And somewhere deep down inside, I wanted the satisfaction of knowing that I had made it, in spite of a lot of small-town people's doubt, skepticism, and disregard for that little girl from the wrong side of the tracks.

And now, against all odds, here I am, with a successful career as an international fashion model. For years, I didn't feel beautiful, but now I do because I know who I am. I didn't give up until I got the life I knew I deserved.

So you see, obviously, my life was not perfect, and my parents and siblings are not perfect, genetically blessed individuals. In fact, if you saw a picture of them, you'd see that none of them has the body of a supermodel.

But I'd like to argue that we are all perfectly blessed, if we can only find our way back to ourselves. If I let my idea of my genetics control my fate, I don't think I'd be where I am today. Neither would my oldest sister, Jena. She was a teenage mother who didn't finish high school, but today, she is one of the best mothers I know, and she'll soon be graduating with a nursing degree.

Our pasts do not determine our fate. We do not have to become our parents. And we do not have to inherit their habits, their lifestyles, their opinions, or their bodies.

I've mastered the Five Keys I mentioned in the Preface and gained self-awareness, and that (rather than weight or hair color or body type or anything else) is what makes me beautiful. Being beautiful isn't about how others see you. It's about how *you* see you. When you feel beautiful, you look beautiful, and then everyone else sees it, too.

MODEL **TALK**

We are not victims of our genes, but masters of our fates, able to create lives overflowing with peace, happiness, and love.

— Bruce H. Lipton, Ph.D., superauthor (from *The Biology of Belief*)

How I Learned Body Love

Like many a model, I get asked all day long the million-dollar question of how I stay so thin. What do I eat? And what exercises do I do? Or do all models actually starve themselves and live off gum and cigarettes? Have I always been thin? Has it *always* been so easy for me?

For as long as I can remember, I have been obsessed with my body. I mean *obsessed!* Like people are today with reality TV. I was that little girl doing Richard Simmons's *Sweating to the Oldies* videos with my mom, or doing crunches, jumping jacks, and push-ups in my bedroom at night. Worst of all, I can't tell you how many times I tried to gag myself with my toothbrush because I was ten and I thought I was fat! I cringe even thinking about how that little-girl me felt so unsatisfied with her body.

Luckily, no matter how far I stuck that toothbrush down my throat, I was never able to throw up my dinner, but I know a lot of girls aren't so lucky. They go down that road. And even if they don't, a lot of young girls share the same body obsession, feeling perpetually dissatisfied with the way they look.

When I signed that first modeling contract several years ago, I wasn't happy with the way I looked. I wasn't as thin as I wanted to be, for one thing. I was almost 20 pounds heavier than I am now, and I had terrible self-esteem. My agents really believed in me, and rather than saying, "You need to lose weight," Nicole Bordeaux, my agent at PhotoGenics, encouraged me to stop lifting weights to help my body become more slender.

I thought she was crazy! I was obsessed with the gym, going there every day for two or three hours, running and lifting weights. I had no concept of how to eat a nutritious meal and practically lived off spinach because I kept reading that it was the healthiest food on the planet. I was hardly eating and was working out all the time, so I thought I was as skinny as I would ever be.

Actually, I was undereating and overdoing it at the gym. The scary reality was that my body thought it was starving, and when I did finally eat, even if it was merely a bowl of spinach, my body would hold on to whatever it could, not knowing when it would get food again. Hello, fat storage! And hello, familiar situation for so many women and girls out there!

FashionSpeak

Most models have agents, and the agent/model relationship is pretty interesting. It can be amazing or it can be terrible, depending on the model, the agent, and the agency. Agents first determine whether they want to work with you, not just based on looks or body, but also on personality. They want to represent models who are different from the models they already represent, and ultimately, they want you to be bankable. In most cases, the better the agent (and agency), the better the jobs, because the best ones have the best clients.

A model may have several agents, but usually has one main agent who controls her (or his) career. This agent decides what jobs to put her up for and what rates to ask for. The agent is the job broker, essentially. The agent is the one who calls up Victoria's Secret and says, "This girl is amazing! Her body is ridiculous. She's absolutely stunning and charming, and there's no one like her! You have to meet her!" If the client agrees, the model gets a casting, or a "go-see," as it's also called. If they like you and want to book you or use you, they call the agent and make the arrangements. They negotiate rates and talk about dates and so on.

The agent also advises the models personally on what to do and not to do, what to wear and not to wear, whether they need to gain weight or, more often, lose weight. A lot of agents send girls to me to help them with their weight, which is how I got started advising people on weight loss. I've been fortunate because I've had agents who really believe in me and treat me like family. This is not always the case. My agents know me better than my own family does, and they really care about me. They work hard for me, and they believe in me. Some agents, however, are rude or mean, and sometimes, they act jealous. They put girls down and make them feel ugly and fat. Unfortunately, there are a lot of those kinds of agents, which does not help the industry.

I took my agent's advice and began eating healthy, regular meals and doing no resistance training. It was ridiculously easy compared to what I was used to, but it worked. Before long, I dropped 20 pounds and I was model-ready, and in no time at all, I was off to New York. From then on, it was a nonstop roller coaster among New York, Milan, and Paris. I made it.

Today I eat more and exercise less than I ever did before I became a model, and have maintained what I believe to be my natural set weight. At 5'10½", I weigh about 117 pounds. Any BMI (body mass index) calculator—and many physicians—will tell you that I am too thin (I'll talk more about the BMI later in this book), but I will tell you with complete honesty that I am healthier and happier than I have ever been. I don't starve myself. I don't throw up (despite those unsuccessful attempts to gag myself with a toothbrush in my youth). I don't take diet pills, and I don't go to the gym every day. I'm at the right weight for me. Not for anybody else, just for me.

I've learned what I love to do and how I love to feel. I do enjoy the gym on occasion, and I especially love yoga class. I'm also a vegan—I don't consume any animal products—and I love raw food. I don't eat this way to make some kind of statement or to stay thin. It's just what makes me feel the best, the most alive, the most energized, and the happiest.

I don't think I have a perfect body. I'm a bit gangly, I've been told I have an alien-looking face (gee, thanks!), and I'm pretty flat-chested. But I love my body! It's all mine. Nobody has a perfect body, but everybody has a body they get to own. I'm finally happy with myself, and I accept every part of me—itty-bitty boobs included!

What Models Know

Of course, we all wish we had the perfect bikini body, but in today's fast-food, sleep-deprived, chemically altered, pesticide-loaded world, sometimes it seems like we have a better chance of getting struck by lightning than of ever getting "model-skinny."

Yet, one group seems to defy nature: *models!* This is why, when I was a young girl, I wanted to be one.

There are a lot of negative stereotypes associated with models and with people who are thin, especially when they are in the spotlight. The modeling industry gets blamed for encouraging eating disorders, and a lot of people point fingers at skinny models, saying that we aren't good role models for women because most women can't ever get the bodies we have.

I don't believe this is true at all. First of all, most of the models I know do not have an eating disorder. Many of them tend to have a tall, thin body type, but not all of them. Kate Moss is only 5'7", and she's one of the most famous supermodels ever.

Second, I believe any woman can have her dream body. Who says you can't get to the weight that makes you feel like a knockout? Telling women they shouldn't want to look good just makes them feel more frustrated, because deep down, they *do* want to look good and feel good. For some women, models are inspirational.

However, it's also really important to remember that fashion models are there to show off clothes, so they often have the bodies that distract least from the way the clothes hang: tall and straight. Your dream body may not be anything like Kate Moss's body, or my body, or Heidi Klum's body, or anybody else's body. But it can be your dream body nevertheless, and that's what I want you to go for.

Don't let anybody tell you that you have to be fat, that you'll always have big hips or a big butt or big thighs. You can have them if you want them, but if you don't want them, you don't have to have them. You can have thin thighs, a tight butt, a flat stomach, and toned arms no matter what body type you have. You can feel good about yourself. You *deserve* to feel good about yourself! Just adopt the Five Keys and watch your dream body materialize. It's really that easy. Love yourself now, but also stay on the path toward where you want to go—and you'll get there.

MODEL **TALK**

Don't let life discourage you; everyone who got where he is had to begin where he was.

— Richard L. Evans, former president of Rotary International and announcer for the Mormon Tabernacle Choir radio broadcast

Why I Wrote This Book

When I first became a model, I thought it would be an amazing opportunity to change the world. I thought: *This is my shot! I'm going to be a <u>supermodel</u>! I'll finally be somebody! I can finally make a difference.*

Since then, I've traveled all over the world for some of the biggest names in fashion. Yet, in all that time, I've never once been asked to speak or write anything. Nobody cared what I had to say. It turned out that it didn't matter how many magazines I shot for, runway shows I walked in, or magazine covers I graced, because I wasn't making a difference in anybody's life. It wasn't what I expected. I thought I would have more power or influence or *something*, in my role as a model. But it was my face and body they wanted, not my ideas. Instead, I was a part of an industry that was potentially harming people and causing eating disorders, low self-esteem, and God only knows what else!

For the longest time, I didn't like to tell people I was a model, because I didn't want to be stereotyped. I was ambivalent about what I did for a living and would joke about being a plumber or cleaning toilets. I realized that saying "I'm a model" came with all kinds of stereotypes and preconceived notions. And then I realized that instead of hiding from the stereotypes, I had an obligation to disprove them. That it was not only important, but that it was necessary.

I could make a difference. I could change the world. But I also realized I was going to have to do it on my own. Then two things happened that made me want to write a book.

The first one had to do with my own family.

I went home my first summer after modeling to see my family, and we went camping on the river. I spent the day swimming, boating, and spending time with my nieces and nephews. The next day, I noticed that my niece wasn't eating. By dinnertime, she still hadn't eaten anything. I asked her why she wasn't eating, and I'll never forget what she said to me: "I'm not eating because I want to be skinny like you, Aunt Sarah!"

She was only eight years old!

This bothered me for a long time, but I wasn't sure what to do about it. Then I entered my first "model apartment."

This was in Paris. I was a new model, and I was living with eight other girls. This is what they do with new models—they put them all together, packed like sardines, into a tiny place where they all have to deal with each other, like it or not.

I shared a room with a really young new model, Bella, from Brazil. She was only 15. She might have even been 14, but you had to be 15 to work in Paris, so her age might have been . . .

exaggerated. She could barely speak English, but we had lots of fun trying to communicate. I've never laughed as hard as I did one day when Bella saw me take a multivitamin and proceeded to ask me if the pill I had just taken was to make me "go"—you know, to keep me skinny. It was hysterical watching this young girl trying to act out taking a laxative! *No, no,* I tried to explain, acting out back to her. *Vitamin. Multivitamin!*

Like so many newbie models, Bella had trouble with her weight because she was so young and didn't know what to eat. This is the age when a lot of girls fall prey to eating disorders, and also when they're dealing with a lot of personal and hormonal issues because they've really just gone through puberty. I watched Bella struggle, trying to balance a young teenager's desire for a lot of food with the pressure of having to stay thin and honestly not knowing how to do it.

I could see my own niece in Bella. Would this be her future? That's when I got the idea for this book. I wanted to help young girls, and women of all ages, to take control of their own lives, to know what foods they need, to know how much they really need to exercise, and to just know themselves. These are the most important keys to getting your dream body and your dream life, and to loving who you are.

This is not a diet-and-exercise book, and I'm not saying you have to be thin to be happy. *Supermodel YOU* is a response to the overwhelming number of questions models get about how we stay thin, and it's a response that is healthy, not dysfunctional. Sadly, a lot of women and girls determine their own value based on their body shape and weight. Self-esteem, self-image, and self-value give rise to your happiness or unhappiness with your body and life, and I realized that this is exactly where I can make a difference. I value my body. I take care of it, feed it, and move it to maintain my positive outlook, and I want every girl and woman to be able to feel this good about themselves. I want them to feel good in their own skin, knowing they are doing the best they can for themselves.

SUPERMODEL **SAYS . . .**

A healthy body at a healthy weight is the best supermodel body. Some models are painfully thin, and that is as undesirable as being overweight. Treat your body with kindness and you'll look great and automatically love yourself more. In the end, it is that love for your own body that gives off those sexy, confident vibrations to everyone. It is really that simple.

— Julia Lescova, superbeautiful Latvian model

It's time to stop picking out all of your flaws in the mirror and declare that today you're on the way to being Supermodel YOU! Although some models are stereotyped as dumb (or just not particularly educated), we definitely know how to look good and feel good about our bodies. We know how to feel beautiful and confident—we are professionals at it. Our bodies are our most prized assets, so we have information to share with you.

But at the same time, every model is different! And every model has a unique body shape. When people try to look like a "model" rather than the best versions of themselves, they can get in a messed-up place, and that's not what true beauty is all about! I don't want to be a role model for disordered eating. I want to be a role model for girls who want to be their own personal versions of supermodels—I want to be a role model for Supermodel YOU! I want you to seek out and find your dream body, but not the one the media brainwashes you into thinking is ideal. Not the body I have, or any other model has. *Your* dream body.

This is what I want for you—not necessarily to become a model, but to feel as confident, sexy, and awesome as models feel. You don't have to be a size 2. If every single girl were a size 2, how boring would that be? Beauty comes in every size, shape, age, and color. What I really want to inspire in you is self-love, self-acceptance, and the energy to take your own body to the place you know it can be. It all starts with a positive shift in your perception, and with the Five Keys I've discovered, which leads to getting the supermodel body of your dreams.

Becoming the supermodel version of yourself has its ups and downs, its easy parts and its challenges, but the Five Keys will help you get there. You are worth the journey and worth the effort, and I don't want you to ever give up on yourself! Never let rejection or fear deter you. Never let somebody else's idea about you hold you back.

Supermodel Gisele Bündchen was rejected by 42 agents at the start of her career when she was just a teenager. Getting "discovered" doesn't guarantee a modeling contract or even an agent, and a lot of agencies told her that her nose was too big. Can you imagine? She says she was finally taken on the 43rd try, and now look at her! She's appeared on countless magazine covers and walked hundreds of fashion runways, and she was the highest-paid model in the world for six years running, making $45 million in 2012, according to *Forbes* magazine. Determination over detour!

MODEL **TALK**

When you get in a tight place and everything goes against you till it seems as though you could not hold on a minute longer, never give up then, for that is just the time and the place the tide will turn.

— Harriet Beecher Stowe, superauthor

The Five Keys

So what are these mysterious keys I keep talking about? These are the five things I've discovered models do to maintain their hot bodies, beautiful faces, and positive attitudes. They are the secrets to becoming Supermodel YOU, and they are what this whole book is based around. The Five Keys themselves are pretty simple:

1. Self-awareness

2. Beauty sleep

3. De-stressing

4. Modercizing

5. Intuitive eating

The practice of them, and how models rock them all, is what you'll learn in these next ten chapters. First, I'll define what it means to be Supermodel YOU. Then I'll talk about energy balance, which is the secret to how models stay so thin. Then, I'll devote a chapter to each key, so you can learn them, memorize them, and begin to feel them in your body and enact them in your life. Finally, I'll provide you with a 20-day plan to start living—and looking—like a supermodel. And in the Appendices, you'll find model meal plans so you can see what models really eat, along with a ton more resources.

MODEL **TALK**

What it takes to be a supermodel is more than beauty and height. Being a supermodel encompasses all things—things like brains, morals, and convictions; and the ability to know your limits and honor your values by how you eat, how you take care of yourself, and how you treat others. The word <u>model</u> means an example, a replica, something to aspire to. If you want to be the perfect example of something, you must work at it and work hard at being your best self and being super on the inside. As a booker for almost 20 years, I can say that those who have staying power in this business use their brains more than their bodies. They are professional, respectful, know their own boundaries and those of others, don't abuse drugs and alcohol, and treat themselves well—and, in turn, their bodies and faces give back to them. And you know, even if you don't fit the physical specifications to be a fashion model, you can still be a supermodel to others in your own way, whether you're a supermom, daughter, sister, friend . . . we are all models to someone!

— Melissa Ghirimoldi, superagent, Muse Model Management, New York

It's easy, it's fun, it's healthier than you might imagine, and you'll get model-skinny and model-pretty in the process.

So forget what you've learned before. Forget diets and workout plans and guilt and self-loathing. You already possess the power to get the body of your dreams. You just need to figure out how to tap into it. The Five Keys are a simple guide any woman or girl can understand, and once you learn the real reasons behind why models are skinny, you'll see how truly easy it is to find your supermodel self, which might be a matter of losing weight or simply accepting the beautiful skin you're already in.

Because if a bunch of models without high school diplomas or genius IQs can get skinny and stay that way, then anybody can. Models can be a great influence on you! Consider us your new clique, and let our behavior rub off on you. Learn the Five Keys and watch your supermodel body emerge without lifting a weight or dropping a fork. It's your birthright. It's your destiny. It's your time.

Now let's rock Supermodel YOU!

■ ■ ■

CHAPTER ONE

What Is
Supermodel YOU?

It's not vanity to feel you have a right to be beautiful.
Women are taught to feel we're not good enough,
that we must live up to someone else's standards.
But my aim is to cherish myself as I am.

— ELLE MACPHERSON, SUPERMODEL, SUPERMOGUL, SUPERACTRESS

Definition of ***Supermodel YOU***

Su·per: Superior. Best. Superb. Outstanding. Exceptional.

Mod·el: A three-dimensional representation of a person or thing, to show the construction or appearance of something. Prototype. Design. Representation.

YOU: YOU!

Description: Aligning with a "super" model version of you to channel your higher self.

Antonyms: Anorexic. Bulimic. Skeletal. One who is skinny by unhealthy means, who is not self-aware, and who does not practice healthy behaviors.

Let's talk about you.

"What?" you might be saying. "I thought this was a book about supermodels! I want to talk about Heidi Klum! And Tyra Banks! And Giselle Bündchen! I don't want to talk about boring old me. I want you to tell me how to look like *those girls!* I want to be somebody! I want you to tell me how to look like *you*, Sarah DeAnna!"

I know exactly how you feel. I used to feel like that, too. I felt like a small-town nobody, and I wanted nothing more than to be one of those beautiful, confident, superfamous supermodels I'd seen in magazines. But I couldn't even imagine it. It seemed totally out of reach to me. How was that ever going to be *me?*

But I've come a long way since then. Not only am I an international fashion model, but I no longer feel like I'm a nobody, or that I can't have the life I want. I know I *can* have the life I want, and it's not because I'm a model. I never would have made it to where I am today if I hadn't believed in myself. I changed my mind, and then I changed my life. And you can, too.

I've got important stuff to tell you—about me, about other models, and about what we know that other people don't . . . other people whose professions don't depend on having great bodies and beautiful faces. But none of it is going to work on you unless we get something straight right now:

You. Are. Beautiful.

Right now. You are fantastic. You are sexy. You are something extraordinary. I am completely knocked out by you. Stunned. Exactly the way you are right *now*. You are gorgeous. And I am totally in love with you—in a platonic way, of course!

I need you to believe every word of that. I need you to start thinking it and telling it to yourself. This is important. This is *crucial*. This is where it all begins. Because if you have somewhere to be—whether you're traveling from, say, Iowa or Kentucky or a small town in Oregon (where I came from) to California, or traveling from your current body to your dream body, or traveling from self-doubt and unhappiness to a life that totally rocks—you have to be all about the self-love. Sing it, sister! You are *amazing*. I mean it! We are in this together, and you totally *rock*. I believe it about you, and I believe it about myself, too. So why shouldn't *you* believe it?

And if you really don't, I want you to do something for me: I want you to fake it 'til you make it. I mean that literally. I want you to fake self-love with so much passion that eventually you're going to convince yourself. Look in the mirror. Forget what you don't like. Look at what you *love.* And if you're not seeing it, just tell yourself (out loud, please—I promise I won't laugh!): "Girl, I am loving your eyes. Your hair is gorgeous. Look at that long neck. Those curvy shoulders. Look at that smokin'-hot butt you've got going on! You are stunning! Adorable! Dazzling! You ooze sex appeal! You totally knock me out!" Just say it. Say it until you mean it.

MODEL **TALK**

It is our attitude at the beginning of a difficult task which, more than anything else, will affect its successful outcome.

— William James, superpsychologist and philosopher

This is the beginning of creating Supermodel YOU, which is about channeling your inner supermodel. Your higher self. It's about becoming the person you want to be, not just physically, but also mentally, emotionally, and spiritually. You know the you I'm talking about.

Here's the good news: You already *are* that person! You just need to unearth her from beneath your false ideas about yourself, your negative thoughts, and your unhealthy habits. And you *should* unearth her. You must! You owe it to yourself to live your best possible life. To be happy, to love yourself, to know that you are truly YOU-nique and be-YOU-tiful—that's what it means to be Supermodel YOU!

You're about to start becoming as good as you can possibly be—and as good as you can possibly be means *perfect!* But my standards for "perfect" may be different from the dictionary's. To me, perfect means to be you in all your natural-born awesomeness. There are a lot of ways to get there, but in this book I'm going to teach you the way I got there, and the way a lot of other models have gotten there. I'm going to give you some model secrets, tricks, and tips to help you in your journey toward the best possible version of yourself. And we're going to get you there together.

This is going to be so much fun! You're going to love getting there. This isn't some deprivation diet or gross, sweaty exercise plan. This is fun. This is about *love,* and dancing, and eating food you love, and giving yourself tons of care and attention. It's about letting yourself be who you are while you move toward who you want to be. It's exciting. It's an adventure.

MODEL **TALK**

I am the greatest. I said that even before I knew I was.

— Muhammad Ali, super–world heavyweight boxing champion

A lot of this is about health. This is a big priority for me. I recently coined the word *skealthy* because I was talking to some people who are totally in the know about weight issues, body-image issues, eating disorders, and all of that. They were concerned about spreading the message that it's good to be *skinny,* and that it can lead girls down an unhealthy path. I get that! As a model, I've seen some girls go down that path, and it's definitely *not pretty.*

In fact, the original title for this book was *Model Skinny,* and while I thought that was a fun title and a lot of people liked it, a lot of other people got prickly about it. They could see how it might mislead. And I totally respected that. So I came up with this new word: *skealthy.* It's even in the Urban Dictionary (**www.urban dictionary.com**). Check it out!

Model Behavior

When you model model behavior, you start to feel more like the Supermodel YOU that you really are! Three ways to do this are to act like a model, think like a model, and know what a model knows.

Acting like a *skealthy* model means doing the smart things models do, like eat! Models eat a lot, and they eat often. They don't really exercise much, but they move all the time and stay active doing the things they love to do. And they also act like they are *hot*. You can totally do that. No acting classes required. This isn't Hollywood . . . but as far as you're concerned, it can be *Hotbodywood!*

Thinking like a *skealthy* model means thinking about who you are and what you do before you do it. Models are self-aware. They don't just shove food into their mouths randomly. They eat what they know will make them feel good, not bad. They don't stay out too late if they know they have an early call in the morning. They make decisions about their behaviors that will maximize their energy and good looks. You can totally do that, too! (But don't think *too* hard. You don't want to hurt your brain! Or suck the fun out of life!)

Finally, *knowing* what *skealthy* models know means understanding how food works in the body, how much you need to move, and what you really want out of your life. You don't have to have a degree in nutrition or sports science. You just need this book and a natural curiosity about life. Learn about what interests you! A lot of models know about a variety of things. Some of them are pretty smart, despite the stereotypes. They learn about things that interest them. A lot of international models speak multiple languages.

You might be wondering why you should listen to me for health advice. After all, I'm not a doctor, a trainer, a nutritionist, or a dietitian. I'm just some "dumb model." Yeah, sure, some models are pretty dumb (or, as I've noted, just not so educated) about certain things, like knowing the capital of Iowa, but one thing we know for sure is how to look good. We have to look good or we're out of a job! And the best way to look good is to *feel good,* and that means cultivating a body that works *for* you, not against you. A body you feel great about. Your dream body!

But how do you do this? I had to know! When I first became a model, I didn't understand why fellow model Katrina was super-skinny even though she ate elaborate home-cooked meals every night, or why 15-year-old Trina, who subsisted solely on sprouts, was being told by our agency to lose weight! But I was fascinated to find out. I was determined to figure out how this could be, because it just seemed so counterintuitive. I observed them like crazy, asked questions, and monitored everything they did. I wrote it all down. I kept notes! I felt like a superscientist!

Here's an example of how I conducted my very "official" supermodel scientific assessment.

Superscientist Sarah DeAnna

I recently did a week's worth of work for Stella McCartney in New York, and I thought this would be an excellent opportunity to fully engross myself in everyone's dietary choices. I prepared my notebook and got myself into observation mode. The crew of people on this particular job included five models, a stylist, five interns, and ten or so Stella employees. I watched what everyone ate, how they acted, how they carried themselves, and how healthy they looked. My theorem: the models would be the experts on how to eat to feel good.

Although I wasn't surprised by the results, you might be: the skinniest girls were the ones who ate the most—me included! We were also the ones with the most energy. We flirted with the boys running the catering, snacked constantly, drank lots of water, and basically ate whatever we wanted all day. If it enticed us, we tried it, but we didn't go crazy and we didn't pig out. It wasn't just me—the other models were doing the same thing.

The rest of the crew, however, was doing something completely different. As is typical during a long day of modeling, we didn't have a real meal until 2 or 3 P.M., and when we did, I noticed that everyone but the models ordered an unhealthy dish—foods that would convert quickly to sugar, like white rice or pasta. The people who hadn't been snacking all day were basically starving by the time lunch arrived. It was fascinating to see which people in our crew needed a jolt of energy and which ones were still going strong.

The models weren't starving because we'd been keeping ourselves well fueled and hydrated via the snack table, so when it was time for lunch, we ordered smartly, ate slowly, enjoyed the food, and saved whatever we didn't finish for later on when we got hungry again.

The other people mostly scarfed down their meals and didn't look like they enjoyed them at all (even though the foods they ordered were supposedly so "decadent"). Then I noticed that most of them suffered a crash a few hours later with a noticeable lack of energy. That's when they started ordering coffee and eating candy.

All the while, ironically, the crew kept complaining about their weight and harassing the models for being "born skinny." It was as if they didn't even notice what was so obvious to me: our habits make us what we are!

The more I see this kind of stuff in action, the more I realize that models really do know a few things about how to have their dream bodies. Models might not know those state capitals or how to do calculus or whatever, but this is a subject we know all about. We are experts, because this is the kind of knowledge that is essential—pretty much a job requirement. Theorem verified!

SUPERMODEL **SAYS . . .**

Put good food into your body. Realize you are what you eat. When you eat that hamburger from the fast-food joint, how do you feel about yourself afterward? Most likely, it's not good. Take control over yourself. No one else will do it for you. Nourish your soul with fresh fruit and veggies. It doesn't get more pure than that. Also, when you do something good, like finally getting to that yoga class you've been trying to do or having your homemade bread turn out perfectly, give yourself a pat on the back. Take in the victory. It creates an anchor and makes you want to feel it over and over again. Most important, though, is to just love yourself. You are you, and that is exactly who you were meant to be. Own it.

— Dani Lundquist, international fashion model

I'm so passionate about how the body works. In another life, maybe I was a biochemist (then I probably *would* have to figure out that whole calculus thing . . .). But if I were a biochemist, I don't know if you would listen to me. My complex science might get boring, and I'm betting I wouldn't be fashion-forward in my white lab coat! But my inner biochemist can't help constantly watching what people eat and how they act, adding up their calorie intakes and thinking about their food choices and how they affect their energy and mental state. I wonder what might be in certain foods to cause this or that effect, and then I research like crazy to find out.

Call me a nerd, but I thrive on that stuff! I do this at breakfast, on the go, at dinner—wherever I am—since I'm so often eating meals with a lot of other people because of my job. I count and observe *everything* from the Happy Meals models sometimes order to the orange juice we swill and breath mints we pop between meals (not at the same time—yuck!). A few years of that, and believe me, I've learned a lot. (Maybe somebody will give me an honorary biochemistry degree! Anyone? Anyone?)

But the thing I notice the most, which blows me away, is the fact that a lot of people who weigh more than I do almost always eat way *less* than I do. Crazy, right? My family is no exception. After a week I spent visiting them in Oregon—and they are all significantly heavier than I am—I observed that they ate less than I did! One day by noon I had already consumed well over 1,200 calories, when most of them hadn't eaten a thing yet.

Here's what else I've figured out: It doesn't take a degree in rocket science to slim down. Most diets work if you stick to them, but most people don't stick to them! Is it because they don't love themselves enough? It is because they don't think it will make a difference? My superwise friend Janice once said to me: "Telling people what not to do has not worked since the beginning of time. Setting examples, educating, and probably most of all, teaching how to find the will to be healthy within themselves is what works. The souls who want to be saved from years of poor choices are the ones who will be able to find the inspiration and knowledge to succeed."

Janice is so right! You just need to want it, to believe it, and to know you deserve it. You don't have to know about science or that the *hypothalamagigger thingy* in your brain regulates how your body functions and how much it wants to eat. (Is that the technical term? Just kidding—you know I mean the hypothalamus, right?) My point is that I may not know that Des Moines is the capital of Iowa without Googling it first (you totally caught me red-handed—thank goodness I'm always glued to my iPhone!), but I'm *skealthy* and I feel great, and according to the people who hire me to model their clothes, I look pretty good, too.

And bear in mind those pictures of models you see in magazines are totally Photoshopped! Nobody really looks like that. In fact, one of Cindy Crawford's most famous quotes is "Even I don't wake up looking like Cindy Crawford." Photos of models in magazines are designed and manipulated for the purpose of showing off clothes or other products. It's marketing, pure and simple, using tools like lighting, camera angles, makeup, particular body positions, and, of course, airbrushing and other special effects. All of these alter how someone looks in a picture. Sometimes, they even crop parts of our bodies to make us look skinnier!

So don't look to magazines for real examples of how you're supposed to look. Look instead to yourself, and what's healthy and right for *you*. That's what models do. We don't care what the photographers do to our images. That's part of the job. But we do care about our real-life bodies, positive attitudes, and having enough energy to do our jobs!

My point is that you can listen to me with confidence because I know this stuff—and you can look just as good as I do, but in your own unique and gorgeous way. Because you are you. And you are about to become Supermodel YOU!

Get ready to make some changes, but nothing that doesn't feel right to you. Get ready to start adjusting your bad habits and morphing them into good ones. Get ready to start eating *more* but *better* food, and get ready to start moving only in the ways that are fun and that you love.

But most important of all, get ready to start changing your attitude and getting to know that cute chick in the mirror. Yes, *you*.

Because it all begins with self-awareness. It's the first and most important of the Five Keys to Supermodel YOU that I'll describe and explain throughout this book. You are the most interesting person you know, no contest. And if you don't know yourself, who will? You've got insider information about yourself. Nobody else can do what you can do to get your dream body and live your dream life.

MODEL **TALK**

Embrace what God gave you! If you are tall, wear heels. If you're petite, embrace small prints on clothes. I was definitely made fun of in school for being tall and skinny. Now it helps me do what I love! Also, find something that makes you happy every day. If you play piano, be the most awesome piano player in your town! If you are great at soccer, practice every day. That's how I've made it. I embraced every activity in life to the fullest. It will help you build a fantastic work ethic that will help you in every area of life!

— Amanda Fields, international model, *Project Runway* model, and guest star on *America's Next Top Model* (@TheRunwayQueen on Twitter)

Your days of making excuses are over. Models see beauty and a great body as their birthright, even if we weren't all born looking like supermodels. We don't sit around making a million excuses for why we're not at the weight we want to be. You'd never hear Heidi Klum or any other model mommy complaining about how she can't lose the baby weight. Heidi Klum doesn't make excuses, because there are none! She knows that our bodies are meant to bounce back, and she and other models *own* their rockin' bodies as part of their very *identity*. That's how people see us, and that's how we see ourselves. Sure, we have our insecure days, but in general, we've made body love a part of ourselves, and it shows.

MODEL **TALK**

I love this quote from Doreen Virtue. Say this to yourself every day and you'll start to believe it, and then it will begin to be true, for real:

You are experiencing positive changes, including your appetite for more whole, organic, fresh, unprocessed, and healthful foods and beverages. You're also drawn toward higher-vibrating relationships and environments.

— Doreen Virtue, superauthor and supermetaphysician

So how do you see yourself? Most people don't say they have the body they really desire. Some people "settle" for taking off ten pounds or whatever, even though the reflection in the mirror isn't what they would really like to see. They "settle" for a life that's less than the one they dream about. Why should you do that? Why should you settle for less than your higher self and your ultimate life? You are the most important thing in your YOU-niverse! Seriously! You can get where you want to go. With a little help from this book, you'll learn how to use your thoughts, your inner words, even that dreaded mirror—and especially the Five Keys—to get the body and life of your dreams. You are a beautiful butterfly wrapped in a cocoon. It's time to break free. It's time to supersede everyone's expectations, time to supercharge your life, time for Supermodel YOU. Let's do it!

■ ■ ■

CHAPTER TWO

Aliens from Planet Model

*When somebody recognizes me, I'm always a little shocked—
like, wait, really? Hang on . . . me? . . . My sisters have always
been these gorgeous glamazons, and I'm, like, this tall, skinny
stick in the family. And I still am the tall girl, even on the
runways. Every time I see Karl Lagerfeld, he's always like,
"Karlie, have you stopped growing yet? Are you taller?" . . .
It used to be something that I really disliked about myself,
being tall and lanky, but it turned out to be the greatest
asset I have—how uniquely weird I am.*

— KARLIE KLOSS, SUPERMODEL (AS QUOTED IN *W* MAGAZINE)

We all know about models, right? They pop Adderall and di-
uretics, smoke like fiends, swallow laxatives, and drink ginormous
amounts of coffee. They all have anorexia or some other eating
disorder. They starve themselves on purpose. They eat apples and
celery, but that's about it. They're supertall, they're superbeautiful, they're supersuperior. They live glamorous lives filled with
travel to exotic locations and tons of money. They're privileged.
They're lucky. They're genetically blessed. They're rich. They drive
expensive cars and wear expensive clothes. They're snobs. They're
skinny, and therefore better than the rest of us.

Right?

Whatever!

Actually, all those assumptions about models are misconceptions, at least most of the time. Since I'm a model, you might assume that I'm vain and brainless and have an eating disorder, that I'm rich and beautiful and turn heads wherever I go—that I'm genetically blessed and I was born on Planet Model, so I'm not like you at all. I wouldn't blame you, because that's what we're all led to believe.

But the simple fact is that it's a lie—the good and the bad. In this chapter, I want to set the record straight. I want you to know what models and the modeling world as I see it are really like. I want you to know who I am and what context I'm coming from, so when I give you advice later in this book—advice on how to get your supermodel body and how to channel your healthy, fit, happy, at-peace, beautiful supermodel self—you feel good about following it. And I don't think you're going to trust me if you think I'm some pill-popping, starvation-obsessed snob with a superiority complex who's going to tell you not to hate me because I'm beautiful.

For one thing, I'm not that beautiful in the conventional sense. I'm actually kind of strange-looking, if you want to know the truth. I was recently asked if my photograph could be part of a new documentary called *Chasing Beauty,* not because I was some perfect example of beauty, but because they wanted an example of an "alien, odd-looking girl." Gee, thanks, guys!

But don't worry. I'm not offended. If I were offended by everything negative I've heard since I became a model, I never would have made it this far. No way would I have the confidence. In fact, I have excellent self-esteem, although it took some work to get it. Learning to spin the negative is all part of what I want to teach you.

But let's get back to the myths, because discovering what's *not* true is part of finally figuring out what *is*.

MODEL MYTH #1:
All Models Are Anorexic, Bulimic, or Have Some Other Eating Disorder

Okay, this one really bothers me, because practically every model I know has, at some point in her life, been accused of having an eating disorder. Let's get real for a minute. This is what happens to you when you have an eating disorder. You get:

- Dry, brittle hair that often falls out

- Dry, cracked nails

- Pale, sallow skin

- Excess body- and facial-hair growth

- Premature aging

- Low energy

- Weakness

- Brittle bones

Does that sound like someone whose business it is to look good? Why would a successful professional model purposely go down this path?

But here's a not-so-happy fact: Eating disorders are the leading cause of death among mental disorders, and the fashion industry and fashion models are the ones we blame more than anyone else for perpetuating them. Eating disorders are serious. They ruin lives. Women are bombarded by images of thin models, and this can result in poor self-image and eating disorders. So it's my fault, isn't it?

I wouldn't be shocked if some readers assumed that I'm not only vain and brainless, but also mentally ill and on a personal quest to destroy society.

But that's not me. And it's not any of the models I know, either.

Still, I understand where the confusion comes in. Girls want to look like models, and they think they have to starve to do it. I'm not a doctor, so I'm not qualified to talk about eating disorders from any official or medical point of view, but if you think you have an eating disorder, please see Appendix C, where I've listed some resources that can help you.

MODEL **TALK**

You are not a mistake. You are not a problem to be solved. But you won't discover this until you are willing to stop banging your head against the wall of shaming and caging and fearing yourself.

— Geneen Roth, superauthor and superexpert on emotional eating
(from *Women, Food, and God*)

Most models don't have eating disorders. And the real problem is the pervasive idea that your body should look like somebody else's body. Whether it's a model, a friend, a movie star, or whoever, it's *her* body. There will be trends in fashion and trends in figures, but when you let them get inside your head, it can really mess you up. You can have the body you desire and still be healthy, but it needs to be *your* dream body, as I've emphasized before.

I'll get into this more later, but for now, let's get back to the misconception that models are doing something wrong.

What's important to understand here is that there is a big difference between being thin and having an eating disorder. I'll tell you another story to make my point. Maybe you've heard of or seen pictures of a supermodel named Chanel Iman. Before she was a supermodel, Chanel and I shared a hotel room in Monterey, California, where we were staying along with about 20 other models flown in for the *Vogue* Council of Fashion Designers of America (CFDA) Fashion Show.

Chanel and I had done a fashion show together in Paris a season or so prior to that, so we knew each other by appearance, but hadn't really ever spoken. I had already been modeling for about a year, and she was just beginning. I remember that she was obsessed with modeling and really wanted to become a supermodel. She was driven and passionate about modeling, and it's no wonder—when your mom names you Chanel Iman, after two great fashion icons, you're destined to do something in this arena.

Chanel kept me up all night asking me about modeling and telling me how badly she wanted to be a star. I told her she would be, with that kind of passion. It didn't take long before she was.

But on that particular trip, before she'd really made it, I remember boarding the bus with the other models to head back to the airport and noticing that Chanel, who was normally super-bubbly and happy, was practically in tears. When I asked her what was wrong, she confessed that the other models were saying bad things about her and accusing her of having an eating disorder.

So even models aren't immune to this mentality, but poor Chanel was extremely upset by this false accusation. Chanel is one of the tiniest girls I've ever seen, but that's just how she's built. She's supernarrow and has no hips at all. She's all legs, arms, and a beautiful smile. But she certainly doesn't have an eating disorder.

In fact, during that trip, she was always eating, and she ate whatever she wanted. She wasn't worried about her food choices, and she definitely wasn't counting calories. She was just eating like a typical teenager. It certainly wasn't a starvation diet. Unlike some of the other girls who were working out and watching what they ate, Chanel was indulging and wasn't hitting the gym at night. That's about as far from an eating disorder as you can get. Chanel is skinny, but she's also healthy, and it's obvious. It's apparent if you just look at her hair, her skin, her eyes, and her energy. That's what many people don't understand. Eating disorders are *not* pretty. Chanel *is* pretty.

Most models get accused of having anorexia, which is a disease where you starve yourself, but bulimia is another ugly and scary disorder. Like anorexia, it can cause hair loss and skin problems, because people with bulimia don't give their bodies time to absorb the nutrients they eat. Bulimia can cause other scary damage, too, like esophageal problems, vocal damage, and dental damage, because people with bulimia binge-eat, then purge their food by vomiting or abusing laxatives. People with bulimia almost always end up with serious swelling. Their faces get rounder and puffier. It's not a way to look good, score a modeling job, or be Supermodel YOU!

According to some recent studies, bulimics end up gaining a lot more weight than people previously believed. In fact, they tend to rebound from any weight loss and often reach the highest weights of their lives. It would be really difficult to be bulimic and maintain a successful modeling career.

But in my experience (and again, of course, I am not a doctor!), people with bulimia have a major problem with self-awareness, which is the first key to Supermodel YOU (see Chapter 4). Self-awareness means tuning in to yourself, so that you know yourself, love yourself, and respect yourself. You have self-esteem, you are even *selfish*, but only in a way that makes you a better person. When you are tuned in to your *self*, you get tuned in to the whole YOU-niverse and you feel great. You know what your body needs, and self-awareness motivates you to *do* what your body needs. Not every model does this, but many of us have found that it has become essential for success in our careers, not to mention in our personal lives.

MODEL **TALK**

I have shot countless young "book-smart" models who have had such a distorted perception of their own bodies, due to their lack of awareness of what a healthy body image really is. Awareness should be a class taught in high schools . . . women in general need to have more awareness of what a healthy body image really is. When you are a model, it's magnified much more. Only when you have a deep awareness will your brain be able to process what is really healthy.

— Greg James, model-turned-superphotographer and model agent

The girls I've known who had bulimia weren't tuned in to themselves or the world around them. I remember one model who was bulimic. Her name was Marla. She was from Poland, and she was such a sweet girl, but she obviously had something wrong with her. For one thing, I noticed that her face and head seemed too big for her body, because her face was always swollen. But even more obviously, she lacked self-awareness. Marla and I shared a model apartment in Milan, and although she was probably the nicest girl there, she was a mess. Whenever she ate, she got food all over her face and clothes, and never seemed to notice. Her zipper was constantly down on her pants, her blouse was often buttoned askew, and her hair was always tangled. Her mental state showed on the outside, and she didn't go very far in the modeling world. She lacked self-awareness, and it showed. It seemed to me that her eating disorder was a dysfunctional way to try to control herself. It obviously wasn't working.

Another side effect of eating disorders and low body weight is infertility, and that's another problem models don't seem to have! Every time I turn around, a supermodel is pregnant! Heidi Klum has four kids; Gisele Bündchen, Adriana Lima, and Alessandra Ambrosio each have given birth to a second child; and Lily Aldridge recently gave birth to her first baby—and that's just to name a few.

So, no—most models are not plagued with eating disorders. Please don't be one of those haters who makes assumptions about models. In general, we are a healthy bunch of girls, and it shows!

There are other reasons why models maintain a lower body weight than the normal population, and they tend to be reasons that result from *healthy* behaviors, not unhealthy ones. This is why I created the term *skealthy*. I'll talk more about how to get *skealthy* throughout the rest of this book.

Modeltude

Most of the models I know *don't* have an eating disorder, but many of them do something kind of strange: they steal food! One of the biggest issues that occur in model apartments is food stealing. It's true! Models will steal and eat other models' food! It's hilarious! And it causes the biggest fights. But to me, it's just evidence that we love to eat, and we eat a lot—not just our own food, but yours, too, thank you very much!

We also often ask to take the food home after jobs, or sneak it into our bags, because sometimes we can't afford to buy our own. (I'll tell you more about the supposed "money" made modeling at the end of this chapter.)

MODEL MYTH #2:
All Models Are as Dumb as a Box of Rocks

Even I'm guilty of poking fun of models' IQs (including my own), but I hope you don't take me too seriously. It's true that a lot of models aren't particularly educated. A lot of them dropped out of school to go into modeling, but the models who aren't book-smart aren't total idiots, either. While your average model might not know the symbol for potassium on the periodic table, models develop another kind of intellect that you can't get from sitting in a classroom. Many of us have traveled the world, speak multiple languages, and know how to deal with people. We know a lot about health and beauty. We know about other cultures and how to get by in the world on limited resources. We're street-smart.

But not at first. A lot of us are from small towns, and our introductions to the big city can make us seem naïve, if not stupid. But innocence is different from stupidity, and the modeling world cures us of our naïveté soon enough.

And although some people like to think that those who are particularly beautiful must have been shorted in other departments and therefore must be stupid, let me point out that a lot of models are not only supersmart, but educated and savvy, too. Who can forget beautiful brainiacs like Cindy Crawford, high school valedictorian; Tyra Banks, who not only started a TV show and production company, but also just graduated from Harvard Business School's Executive Education Program; and supermodel/supermogul Kathy Ireland, whose company is worth over a billion dollars and who was pictured on a 2012 cover of *Forbes* magazine?

So yes, sure, I'm going to joke a little about the stereotypes sometimes, but let's agree that being a model is *not* evidence of a lack of intelligence. "Model" is a job title, not an IQ score.

SUPERMODEL **SAYS . . .**

If there is one thing I can say about my modeling experience, it's that it has been an extreme and accelerated education in self-management. The very nature of a modeling career involves being a canvas for projections of art and beauty. Being part of the creative process is totally exciting, but when girls (and guys!) mix up the "blank canvas" concept with their lives outside of work, that's when the problems start. For instance, as a model, you will hear a lot of people's opinions on how you should eat and exercise, what parties to go to, which agency to switch to, which creepy photographer to avoid . . . the list goes on and on. I've been told by models and clients that smoking and cocaine are great for losing weight. I was told by an agent one day that I needed a nose job, and the next day told by a photographer that I had the most beautifully straight Indian nose that he had ever seen!

This is where my small-town upbringing came to the rescue for me. Everyone is going to have an opinion. It's part of the job. After all, you are a "model" for concepts, ideas, emotions. But the key is to always maintain the intention and heart that you had when you walked onto that first runway. For me, the core of that intention was always to push myself to be the best that I could be, but never to take a job or listen to input that required me to disrespect myself or others. One of my favorite female leaders, Eleanor Roosevelt, once said, "No one can make you feel inferior without your consent." It's a widely known phrase, but I remind myself of this every day as a model.

The first day that I decided to walk down a runway—not focusing on my straight head or swingy arms or yada, yada, yada, but instead, just thinking about how badass it is that no matter what they put on me to wear, my same strong, loving, goofy spirit would shine through—was the first day of a storm of consistent bookings that hasn't stopped yet.

— Natasha Lannin (aka "Asha"), supersmart, supergorgeous
model and UCLA graduate, represented by
L.A. Models Runway/PhotoGenics

Model Myth #3:
All Models Are Drop-Dead Gorgeous

The fashion designer Diane von Furstenberg once said: "A lot of fashion models are more strange-looking than beautiful. Most of the successful catwalk models are not very beautiful when you see them in real life. They are often quite odd-looking."

I love that quote! And I'm pretty sure she was talking about girls like me. As I mentioned before, I'm not your typical "beauty." The modeling industry has placed me in the strange, exotic, edgy, weird-girl category. About 99 percent of the time, my hair is slicked back, I look like a dude, and I'm told under no circumstances to smile! God forbid I might look happy.

But it's true that people who don't necessarily look classically beautiful are often more in demand as models because they look unusual and they stand out. And the better-looking a model is, male or female, the less interesting that individual seems to be to designers and photographers. It's funny! They don't like that typical kind of perfection. They like to take something not generally considered beautiful and make it beautiful. It's a challenge.

Many of us have moles, acne, cellulite, or some body part that looks too big or too small when compared to "normal" (whatever that means). We have all kinds of other "imperfections," but those are what make us unique and special, and I think that's just a different kind of perfection. When I was recently shooting with Heidi Klum for her new shoe line, she candidly joked with famous photographer Rankin about not catching her lazy eye! She was laughing and kidding around about it, and I thought that was so adorable! I loved it. This is what it means to be confident and to spin the negative into something light and funny that makes you feel good about yourself instead of bad.

MODEL **TALK**

To feel like a supermodel, you must face yourself, forgive your-self, and above all, <u>love yourself.</u> Real beauty is something that radiates from within.

— John Tew, super–celebrity beauty guru (**www.beauteguru.com**)

When I first started modeling, I was always surprised when I'd meet girls who were doing really well in fashion. The girls who were getting *Vogue* covers and campaigns were always the last girls I would've expected to do so. Meanwhile, the girls I thought were the most gorgeous struggled to get jobs.

One of the first models I shared an apartment with in Milan was this ridiculously beautiful Romanian girl. She was well over six feet tall and absolutely stunning. She had piercing blue eyes, beautiful full lips, and a perfect body. She worked enough, but she also struggled to rise to that supermodel level, because she was (and still is) just "too beautiful," according to industry standards.

We ended up sharing a model apartment in Paris for a while, too, and became close friends. Once I started booking big jobs, I remember saying to her how awesome it would be to shoot to-gether. I'll never forget what she said to me:

"Oh, you and I, we will never shoot together. I'm much too beautiful, and you are, well . . . you are high-fashion and edgy."

At the time, that hurt my feelings, but I get it now. I'm not the classic beautiful girl. I'm different. My look is strong. My fea-tures are strong. I have huge green eyes, superhigh cheekbones, and a very pronounced bone structure. She, on the other hand, is beautiful, flawless, soft, and what is called *commercial*. Being com-mercial means your look is more common and likable—the "girl-next-door" look. Being *editorial* means your look is typically more interesting, if not necessarily beautiful. My model friend wasn't trying to offend me or put herself above me. She was just observ-ing that we were in different categories of beauty. She was com-mercial. I was editorial.

FashionSpeak

A *commercial* look is the all-American look that appeals to the masses. An *editorial* look is a unique look that appeals to a smaller demographic within the high-fashion community. You can see the commercial look in advertisements for stores and brands like Target and Old Navy, and the less-expensive-product advertising for skin care, hair care, and toothpaste. You'll also be more likely to see the commercial look on television ads. You're more likely to see the editorial look in ads for brands like Gucci, Dior, and Calvin Klein; in ads for expensive skin-care products; and in magazines like *Vogue*. Sometimes there will be crossover.

These days, the Victoria's Secret and *Sports Illustrated* models tend to have a more commercial look. This is just a general description, however. There are often exceptions, like a more commercial look in a high-fashion ad, or an editorial look popping up occasionally in an ad for a more mainstream brand. There are also those models who can look commercial or editorial, depending on how they are made up.

Here's another example of how not all models are unusually beautiful. A few years ago, I was in Tokyo on a modeling contract. That's how they do it there—you get a contract, and you go for a few weeks to a few months. They put me and the other models up in a hotel, which was unusual. Typically we would be in an apartment with girls from our agency only, but in this case, the hotel housed a mix of models as well as American students who were studying architecture at the university in Tokyo, and many of them were boys. Naturally, the girls and the boys would hang out together. I asked the guys if this was their dream living situation—to be in a hotel with a bunch of models. They all surprised us with their answer. They said there were just as many beautiful girls back home on campus as in our hotel.

I loved that! It just further proved my theory that models aren't any more beautiful than anybody else. We are all beautiful!

SUPERMODEL **SAYS . . .**

Beauty starts from <u>within.</u> Many people have this warped view that beauty is characterized by what you look like on the outside. It's <u>not.</u> I feel confident just putting on mascara, a little blush, and ChapStick. Believe, love, speak <u>life,</u> and have faith in yourself. It has taken me a long time to realize what true beauty is. As you get older, looks do fade, but it's how you believe in yourself, and how you have faith in your abilities, that makes you a true supermodel.

— Candice Carruth, super-sunshine model (she's always smiling!), represented by Muse Model Management, New York

MODEL MYTH #4:
All Models Are Superskinny

There are tons of clients out there, each with their own concept of an ideal body. That means there are modeling jobs for women of all shapes and sizes. Lara Stone, one of the most popular high-fashion models of the moment, is a size 6 or 8, depending on your source, even though high-fashion models are typically a size 2 or 4. Crystal Renn, another hottie model, has a beautiful, sexy, strong body, even though she has done plus-size modeling (in the fashion industry, "plus size" can be as small as a size 6 or 8!).

The only reason models are usually skinny in the first place is because fashion samples are small. Designers don't work on bigger mannequins. I'm not sure why, but some people say it's because mannequins are still the same size they were when they were invented hundreds of years ago, and back then, women were smaller. It's true that since the 18th century, the average sizes for women and men have increased. We're all taller, and we weigh more. We have changed, while mannequins have not.

Part of it also might be that working on small mannequins saves money because it requires less fabric and material. Models have to fit these samples. And of course, designers want people to notice the clothes, not the models' bodies, so the more we wear clothes in the way they would look on a coat hanger, the more the designers like it. Clothes hang a certain way on tall, thin bodies. Those kinds of figures don't steal the focus from the clothes.

Still, not all models are superskinny or supertall. The use of superskinny models is most prevalent in couture modeling, but both Jean Paul Gaultier and John Galliano recently used so-called plus-size models in their shows.

Honestly, a lot of models don't do the couture shows because they can't fit into the clothes. Their frames are too big! Even some of the thinnest girls can't fit into the clothes because of their particular bone structure. Couture modeling traditionally requires a very specific kind of figure. A girl can have twigs for arms and legs, but unless she breaks a few ribs and shaves her hips, she's not going to fit into that couture gown.

So much of it is a matter of proportion, and also of perception. I can actually fit into a lot of those couture gowns just because of my proportions, but when people see me, they often say things like "Oh yeah, you look healthy; you're not that skinny." And it's true. Any particular modeling job will have very specific requirements for frame type, and that has nothing to do with "skinny" or "plus-size" or any other adjective to describe a woman's shape or size. I can look larger than a girl who can't fit into the dress size that I wear. Once, I could fit into an Oscar de la Renta dress they couldn't even squeeze onto the mannequin!

That's because models, just like any other woman, come in all shapes and sizes. That says nothing about beauty or health or how someone feels in her own skin, all of which have nothing to do with the particular profession of modeling.

MODEL **TALK**

The reason we struggle with insecurity is because we compare our behind-the-scenes with everyone else's highlight reel.

— Steven Furtick, superinspirational pastor

Model Myth #5:
All Models Are Genetically Blessed
or Luckier Than the Rest of Us

If you read the Introduction, you already know that I was far from genetically blessed and had an underprivileged and dysfunctional childhood. A lot of models are from small towns and have had pretty hard childhoods, come from families who have a lot of problems, or have overweight relatives.

The notion that genes determine one's body, personality, and life is just a crazy belief we've all been fed and keep feeding ourselves. It manifests itself in so many ways, large and small. I used to believe that I would always have "thunder thighs," because that's what my mom always said and believed to be true about herself. But I was wrong! I don't have thunder thighs anymore, because I took control of my genes and changed my environment and habits and my life.

Of course, genetics does play a role. It can predispose you to things. It can make you susceptible. But it doesn't doom you. And if there are traits you can't change, then change what you *can:* your attitude about them.

For example, I always thought that I had "big bones" and was therefore a "big girl." But what does that mean? I realized, once I was out on my own and learning about body types and nutrition, that I'm not big-boned at all. I'm tall, but my frame is tiny, and there was certainly no reason at all for me to be overweight, even though a lot of people in my family are on the heavier side.

But what about my ginormous *man hands?* What was I supposed to do about them? You can't change your hand size through lifestyle choices. So I changed my attitude. I used to hate my hands . . . until I realized I could palm a basketball and throw a perfect spiral football better than most boys I knew!

And that was empowering.

SUPERMODEL **SAYS . . .**

It sounds so clichéd and corny, but you have to love yourself. You have to be kind to yourself. You have to focus on your strengths. Spend time with yourself. Be proud of who you are. Love your body because it's healthy and it works. Appreciate what you have. Don't like your thighs? Why? Do they not work? Do they not move you from place to place? What would you give for your legs if you didn't have them? Count your blessings; find a way to do this. If you can't, get someone to help you. There's no shame in getting a therapist. Everyone in New York City has one. Have you ever seen someone in love? How gorgeous. Find a way to love yourself and you will shine. Then, get a really hot boyfriend for . . . ahem . . . exercise.

— Audi Martel, supermodel, supermusician
(singer in Le Blonde), superwriter

MODEL MYTH #6:
All Models Are Supertall

A willowy six-foot-tall woman—isn't that the supermodel stereotype? Actually, a lot of models lose jobs because they're too tall. If you're too tall, the clothes don't fit right. There are some ridiculous fashion trends at times, but high-water pants aren't one of them, and neither are shirts that unintentionally show your midriff or skirts that don't fall in the right place over your hips because you're too long-waisted. Plus, if you're shooting a commercial and you're extremely tall, chances are you're taller than the rest of the talent, and then it doesn't look right. You can't be towering above everybody else. It's distracting. Or you make the product look too small.

What's more, if you're tall, chances are your feet are huge, too. You need big feet to balance that tall body properly, but that's not helpful for fashion shoots. Most tall models wear a size-9 shoe, but if you're pushing six feet, your feet are going to be bigger, probably size 10 or 11, or even larger. Not many shoes are made that big.

Kristy, one of my really good model friends, is about six feet tall, and I'd guess her feet are a size 11. Often, she can't fit the footwear. If she can, she will cram her poor little toes into too-small shoes and suffer the pain, but sometimes it's just not possible. And that means she can't do the job.

Shoe samples, like clothing samples, tend to be small, usually a size 7. That means shoe models are generally short. Whenever I do "market" for Stella McCartney, they book a girl named Elizabeth who is an actress/parts model. She is only 5′6″, but she fits the shoes and she's beautiful. And she sells those Stella shoes!

FashionSpeak

After a fashion show, a collection goes to market. The way this happens is that designers set up showrooms, usually specific to the clients, typically at their headquarters. Buyers come from boutiques and stores like Neiman Marcus and Saks. Market is the first time the buyers can see the collections up close. The designers hire models to walk around showing the clothes.

For a model, this can be a job from hell or a really great gig, depending on the situation, the client, the designer, and the terms. It typically involves crazy-long hours; changing clothes about a thousand times; and a lot of walking, standing, and wearing high heels. It's not glamorous, but it pays well, depending on how much you do and on the work conditions. You might be treated really well, or you might be stuffed into a closet with ten people.

Clients who are really tuned in to their target market will also use samples and models to best represent their brand. Bebe, for example, uses models who are a size 4 to 6, not size 2. I don't often work for Bebe because of this, with the exception of their runway shows, because most designers use thinner/smaller runway models. I don't know why that is, although it's not set in stone, either. Like I said before, Galliano has used plus-size models on his runway, and Lara Stone and a few other "bigger" models—and by bigger, I mean bigger than size 2—are still killing it on the runway.

Ultimately, getting the gig depends on the brand and the cut of the line of clothes, and of course, on the model—not just her size, but also her look, her energy, and her behavior. The models who stand out more tend to be the ones who succeed, just like the people who stand out tend to be the ones who succeed at anything in life. I firmly believe that if someone, anyone, truly wanted to model because they really loved it, they could do it, regardless of what they look like or what size they are. If you pursue modeling as a passion, you will be successful (but as you'll see later in this chapter, it might not be the career you thought it was).

But back to height. Heather Chantal Jones, a runner-up on *America's Next Top Model,* once said: "I'm a flippin' giant, probably six feet. That's too tall!" As for me, I'm just shy of 5'11", and whenever I go on a commercial casting assignment, my agent always tells me to wear flats.

Models who are too tall have a particularly hard time in Japan and other Asian countries because the general population is shorter than in the U.S. Most of the really successful international models are closer to 5'8" or 5'9" than to 5'11". Many of them are even shorter.

So forget that stereotype. As I mentioned, Kate Moss, one of the most famous models in the world, is only 5'7". Twiggy, one of the first supermodels, was only 5'6". Anyway, the stereotype may be about to change. Recent research by a modeling agent named Ben Barry showed that consumers were more likely to buy clothes from brands that market to them. The study of 2,500 women in a range of ages and sizes proved that women were more inclined to pay a high price for a Diane von Furstenberg wrap dress if they saw it modeled on a woman with a figure resembling their own rather than on a skinny model. I think this is significant, and maybe even a sign that women are beginning to accept their own bodies more. Hooray! I believe over time, we're going to start seeing a huge transition in model bodies and looks.

MODEL **TALK**

My first piece of advice to give to any model would be to listen. Listen to your agents. Listen to your managers. Most importantly, listen to your body. In order to be successful in this industry and truly have a remarkable career, you must not only take the guidance of your agency, but also be aware of your mind, body, and soul. The agency can only take you so far if you are not well grounded and aware of what you are doing with yourself. It is important to eat healthfully and exercise not just the body, but your mind as well. Doing anything that will be detrimental to either part of you will surely be the start of the end of your career.

— Phira Luon, supermodel agent, scout, and one of
my personal superbookers at PhotoGenics

MODEL MYTH #7:
All Models Work Out Constantly

I have to be honest with you here: Some models are the laziest people on the planet! Sure, some of them work out or love to go running or do yoga, but even the ones who hate to work out burn plenty of calories and get plenty of exercise, often without ever going to the gym. You probably get plenty of exercise, too, in your daily life. You just might not know it.

For one thing—and this might surprise you—"exercise" is in your head. I recently read about the coolest study, conducted in 2008 by Harvard psychologist Ellen Langer. She was studying hotel maids, who have very rigorous jobs that require a lot of physical activity. Yet, when she interviewed the maids, most of them said they didn't get any exercise. Their percentage body fat, waist-to-hip ratio, blood pressure, body mass index, and weight all reflected this—they had the bodies of people who didn't exercise, even though they *did* exercise.

So Langer decided to figure out if the effect was mental. She divided the housekeepers into two groups. She informed one group about how many calories they were actually burning while doing their jobs, how much exercise they were already getting, and how they were already meeting the standard for an "active lifestyle." The other group was given no information.

After just one month, Langer interviewed all the housekeepers again. None of them reported changing anything about what they actually did, and the hotel that employed them agreed there had been no changes in how any of the work was being performed. Even so, the group of housekeepers who had been told how much exercise they were getting showed significant decreases in blood pressure, weight, and waist-to-hip ratio. Just knowing they were exercising changed how their bodies responded to the exercise. The group given no information showed no changes at all.

The key was awareness! And this is also the first key to being Supermodel YOU, as you'll read later.

My point is that you don't have to live at the gym or even do anything differently than you are doing now in order to get enough exercise. If you clean your own house, walk the dog, cook food from scratch, run around after your kids, go out dancing with your friends, go shopping, do a few sit-ups and push-ups, or just fold laundry when you watch TV at night, *it all counts.* When you move your body, you are exercising. The average person burns 224 calories an hour by simply mopping the floor. This is not that different from running on a treadmill for the same amount of time.

The models I know get most of their exercise by going dancing, shopping, or just running around on the job. The trick is that they *think they are getting enough exercise.* Models always complain about how much they have to move. And they really appreciate it when they don't have to. Moving = exercise. Not moving = relaxation. That's a pretty healthy attitude.

I have to admit that I really enjoy working out, and I probably always will. I've always loved the rush I get from a good workout. I even enjoy going to the gym. It's my time alone with myself. I usually don't talk to anybody because I need that time to recharge and work my muscles. It makes me feel balanced.

But I'm not lifting heavy weights or killing myself on a treadmill. Boring! Instead, I love doing anything active, like sports, yoga, hiking, and walking. And I need it! I relieve a lot of stress at the gym, especially in yoga class.

But I also move my body in a lot of other ways. I love to clean (weird, right?), and I burn tons of calories scrubbing my floors. I also love to get outside. I have so much fun playing beach volleyball. I'm also a big fan of spin class—but not just any spin class. I think my spin instructor, PK, is the best in the world. He has a huge following, and all of his classes are packed because he's fun. He plays the best music, which makes it feel more like a dance club than a gym class. He even brings black lights and other colored lights, and we seriously rock out while working out. I absolutely love it! And I go to yoga because it's fun, but also because it calms me and keeps my stress in check. One of my favorite yoga instructors, Jennifer Pastiloff, does Karaoke Yoga—a trendy new form of yoga in Los Angeles where you sing and dance while you do yoga—which she invented. She even has a DJ doing the music!

The physical benefits of all this movement (more tone, more muscle mass, and so forth) are a bonus, as are the other great perks, like less stress, improved self-confidence, and so on. That's what makes it all feel like fun, rather than a workout. And that's the key to the way models exercise (or *modercize,* as I like to call it). Doing what you love is the key to a successful exercise regimen.

You don't have to exercise at the gym to get enough movement in your life, just like you don't have give up carbs, meat, or anything else to have a supermodel body, unless you really want to and feel like it's right for you. What's important is doing what you love! Eating what you love!

MODEL MYTH #8:
Modeling Is <u>So</u> Glamorous

On *America's Next Top Model,* Tyra Banks houses girls in amazing spaces for the sake of "reality TV," but I'm here to tell you that is not reality at all.

Let's start with the model apartment in New York City where I lived with a group of other models. One of the biggest and most prestigious agencies provided us with these living quarters, for which we each had to shell out $1,200 per month in rent. Was it glamorous?

Luxurious? Hardly. This place was a rat-infested crap hole, a dirty one-room dump with a teeny-tiny bathroom. Models would come and go, in and out of the model apartment, according to their jobs, and they would crash anywhere they could. It wasn't pretty. At the time, my agent told me that it was the same apartment where Kate Moss and all the other really famous models once stayed, as if this would be incentive for me not to complain about it!

I'll never forget one of my worst modeling days. I got out of bed that morning in that dumpy apartment after not sleeping because a crazy Russian girl was up yakking on the phone while another model was sick and coughing all night. I had to take the subway in the freezing cold to my job. When I arrived on the set, I discovered the heat in the building was broken. This was the middle of winter. I think it was something like six degrees outside, and maybe even colder inside.

I spent the day ingesting hair spray, which made my nose hairs stick together. I had an allergic reaction to some makeup product. I was poked, pushed, and teased for hours. And then I had to try to look pretty in sultry summer clothes, even though I was shaking so badly from the cold that my skin was turning white and I felt like I was having convulsions. At the end of the shoot, I hit rock bottom when I had to ask to take home some of the leftover lunch and snacks because I was too broke to buy food.

Yep, pretty glamorous. And don't even get me started on the little things, like feet, and how most models end up with the gnarliest, jacked-up, most disgusting toes you will ever see, from being crammed into countless ridiculously uncomfortable shoes.

Jealous yet?

MODEL MYTH #9:
All Models Live a Life of Sex, Drugs, and Partying

Okay, I need to clear up some major misconceptions about this one. Let's start with sex. Most models are really young, and have often never even kissed a boy. Anja, a model friend of mine, started working when she was 14, and by the time she was 20, she *still* had never kissed a boy.

Drugs and alcohol? I've heard a lot about the old supermodel era and drugs, but models doing drugs is *so* 20th century. Just because I'm a model, people think I do them. It's comical! In fact, I'll never forget being at a party a few years ago in Hollywood. This girl approached me and asked if I wanted to do blow. I thought she was trying to recruit me for some kinky sexual fantasy, or that maybe she was challenging me to a bubble-gum-blowing contest! I seriously had no idea what she was talking about. I certainly wouldn't have guessed that "blow" meant cocaine. She probably didn't know what to think of me, but in retrospect, *I* think it was pretty hilarious.

Recently, I got a text from a guy friend that said: "I have Molly if you want to try tonight." Again, I was like, *Huh?* I thought maybe he sent it to the wrong person, like he meant to text another guy because he was obviously referring to a girl named Molly, and maybe he was gearing up for a threesome? Geez, I must have a perverted mind! But then I found out that "Molly" is a code name for MDMA, which is the purest form of the drug ecstasy. Ha, what do I know? Actually, I'm pretty proud that I *didn't* know!

A few models might do drugs, but they aren't going to last very long in the business if that's their priority. Because the fact is that if you do drugs, it's going to show on the surface. Not only do models have to look good, but they also have to be super-responsible. Models have early call times, flights to catch, places to be. That's not conducive to a life full of benders and hangovers.

Most models don't drink a lot, either. Alcohol has a ton of empty calories, excess sugar, and a bunch of ugly side effects. Empty calories cause the wrong kind of weight gain, and excess sugar leads to breakouts, accelerated aging, sleep interruptions (see Key 2), stress (see Key 3), bloating, and worse. No self-respecting or halfway ambitious model would allow that.

And as for smoking, in my experience, cigarettes are no more prevalent among models than they are among the rest of the population. Some people smoke, but more and more don't. I'd even venture to say models smoke less than the general population. Smokers aren't going to land any makeup campaigns or major magazine spreads. Even the best digital retouching couldn't gloss over the fact that you've got yellow teeth and gray skin. Smoking is just not pretty.

Finally, let's talk about the party-animal myth. *Please.* Most models don't party! Don't get me wrong: we like to go out, and we love to dance—that's our exercise—but we're not staying up all night closing the clubs and then working the after-parties. Models know they need their beauty sleep (again, see Key 2). Not only does alcohol interfere with your beauty sleep, but it also makes you bloated and puffy, which is totally *not* Supermodel YOU. So sleep deprivation plus alcohol is a bad combination.

Maybe these rumors about the wild model lifestyle are all products of a past era, but I'm telling you what the modeling world is like *today,* and we are more likely to be fresh, clean, healthy, well rested, properly nourished, and ready to rock the runway or the photo shoot.

SUPERMODEL **SAYS . . .**

Respect yourself before expecting anyone else to respect you.

— Jarah Mariano, supergorgeous *Sports Illustrated* and Victoria's Secret supermodel, represented by IMG Models
(**www.officialjarahmariano.com**)

MODEL MYTH #10:
All Models Are Self-Centered and Stuck-up

I'm not going to lie here: some models *do* have major attitude. But I'd say they are the minority. What some people might interpret as acting stuck-up is often just a front for maintaining sanity while your looks are being scrutinized and judged on a daily basis, often by nasty, rude industry people who don't show models respect. It's self-protective. We have to go inside our shells a little, and you wouldn't blame us if you heard how rude these people can be sometimes, for no apparent reason. Whether it's an agent, a photographer, a casting director, a makeup artist, a hairdresser, or anyone else in the industry, some of them are nice and some are just incredibly nasty, personally attacking our looks, body, walk, or whatever.

If you want to work in this business, you have to be prepared for this and have some strategies to help you deal with it so you don't take it seriously. We prepare as well as we can for jobs, and we put up with the rudeness because the benefits of the job are worth the effort of ignoring the negatives. Something that one person hates might be the very thing that wins you a job the next day, but you really have to stay centered and positive, and let the negatives bounce off. It can be confusing and a total mind game, and sometimes the way models respond is to put up a protective shell. And sometimes, it gets to them.

This makes me think of Camilla. I first met Camilla in Paris during Fashion Week. I was immediately intimidated by her—and so was everyone, because she was drop-dead gorgeous and she knew it. She was also a total b*%ch! She had a way of making everyone around her feel small and insignificant.

When she first started modeling, everyone who saw her wanted to shoot her and work with her. Photographers and casting directors would fall all over her, and she got a lot of great bookings, but here's the important part: she never got rebooked. She had such a diva attitude that nobody wanted to work with her a second time. Beautiful or not, her looks were less important than her attitude for making it in the business. Later, I learned that this was just her way of dealing with her own insecurities, but that excuse didn't help her career. She let modeling get to her, and it turned her into someone nobody wanted to work with.

My agent in Paris always said modeling is so much more about your personality than your looks. He was totally right. If people don't like you, they will rarely rebook you, no matter how gorgeous you are. This is true for actors, too. Actors are often cast in multiple films by the same director, based on their personalities. Think about directors like Woody Allen and James Cameron. You see the same actors in their movies again and again.

Models get rebooked by photographers, magazines, and brands when they are easy to work with. Needless to say, Camilla never works in Paris anymore because she burned too many bridges there, but it was refreshing to run into her recently in New York and see that she had changed a lot.

By the way, I think this is relevant for any job or just for getting along in the world. Why be a diva when you can be a human being?

SUPERMODEL **SAYS . . .**

Supermodels stand out from the rest of the beautiful girls because they glow, and that comes from the joy of being yourself.

— Bianca Warren, super-*bonita* model,
represented by Ford Models, New York

MODEL MYTH #11:
All Models Make a Lot of Money

Don't make me laugh! Many models live off a stipend that averages out to about $200 a week, especially in their first year of modeling. We'd make a lot more working at a coffee shop. With that kind of money, models can barely afford to eat and get around in cities like New York, Milan, or Paris, where many jobs take place. In fact, many models drive clunkers (if they can afford a car at all) and shop at thrift stores, vintage stores, and cheaper re-tailers like H&M and Forever 21, because that's all they can afford.

But here's one of the ways I think models get it right. Some-how, despite their budgets, they make their clothes look hot. They pull it off. Instead of bemoaning the fact that they can't buy ex-pensive clothes and cars, models tend to pride themselves on find-ing cool outfits that cost next to nothing. They'll think: *This is a total steal* or *This dress looks exactly like the one Dior did* or *This old beater-mobile gets great gas mileage. I'm so eco-chic!* They may not be rich, but they tend to have good taste.

To be honest, if I hadn't actually believed the myth that models make a ton of money, I probably never would've started modeling. I, too, thought models made millions of dollars. In truth, very few make enough to even support themselves without taking a second job. Many models are also bartenders, waitresses, and so on, just as it is with actors. Only the ones whose careers really take off can afford to quit their "regular" jobs. I never took a second job because I was too proud and wanted to prove I didn't need one, but I really dug myself into a financial hole when I first started modeling.

In some ways, modeling is actually worse than acting in terms of income, because unlike with acting, there is no union or law governing our income. We have no benefits, no protections, no regulation, no minimum wage, not even mandatory lunches and breaks. According to sociologist Ashley Mears in *Pricing Beauty: The Making of a Fashion Model,* the median income for a model in the U.S. in 2009 was $27,330—and, as I mentioned, that's with no benefits.

Plus, sometimes we don't get paid at all! Models often work for free or get paid in trade with clothes. It's ridiculous, but it just shows how many people don't respect what we do. A lot of designers don't pay models for their shows or pay very little because they claim it's publicity for the model. The same is true of magazines. Even covers. Yep, magazine work, called *editorials* in the industry, doesn't pay or pays very little.

FashionSpeak

Editorials are compilations of photos published in magazines that tell a story rather than obviously endorsing a product. When a look is *editorial,* as defined earlier, that means it is good for fashion-magazine editorials.

Ironically, these are some of the most coveted jobs. How backwards is that? They expect us to be grateful for the exposure, but they don't think we should expect actual money. (My writer, painter, and musician friends tell me it's similar for them—people think they should be happy to create their work for free as long as they are getting exposure. Exposure doesn't pay the rent, people!)

In my first year of modeling, I didn't make a dime. Sure, I booked plenty of jobs, including magazine covers, major runway shows, and even *Italian Vogue,* the crème de la crème of modeling jobs. But after agency fees, plane tickets, and all the other expenses, I seriously took home nothing. How did I survive? I borrowed money. I racked up major credit-card debt. I would take food home after shoots and jobs. I squeaked by.

The worst part was later learning that I actually could have made money, but my agency wouldn't book the money jobs. Apparently, Macy's, Target, and several other companies wanted to book me, but my agency felt the jobs weren't prestigious enough. You have little or no say at all in where your agency books you, especially when you first start modeling, but I thought this was absurd. I couldn't afford to pay my bills and buy food, and they were telling Michael Kors they couldn't have me because the client wanted me to do showroom and my agency preferred they book me for their campaign? It was harsh. Now that I'm more established in my career, I have more input on where and how I get booked, but not in those days.

FashionSpeak

A *campaign* is the whole plan for a company's advertising, including how they will brand their images used for promotion. To be booked for a company's campaign means they will use you in their branding images.

A *showroom* is the location where samples of a designer's latest collection are showcased.

While I now understand what my agency was doing, and it was flattering that they believed so much in my future career, being broke was a huge stress on me during my first year or so of modeling. I felt that just because I grew up poor and on public assistance, was teased for being a "welfare baby," and didn't have the clothes and shoes the other kids got to wear, it didn't mean I was destined to be poor. I refused to be! But there I was—digging myself into a bigger and bigger hole, shooting for some of the biggest magazines and covers, yet not being able to afford to eat. It was ridiculous.

This was also hard on me because I'd made damn sure I had a good education so I could make money. I'd studied so hard and was always an overachiever, so not having enough money really hurt my ego. This wasn't what I'd planned for myself, what I'd *promised* myself! At the same time, I was still learning the ropes in modeling and was still in the process of building my self-esteem. That was a really hard time in my life, realizing that success would require even more work—much, much more work—than I'd already put in trying to improve my life. It was a harsh lesson.

The whole industry is a total psychological manipulation. Luckily for me, I walked away from the game when I needed to. Sure, maybe if I had stuck it out longer, I'd be shooting for Victoria's Secret or *Sports Illustrated* or whomever right now, but it wasn't worth it for me to be manipulated that way. What the fashion industry does, essentially, is tear the models so far down that they have no ego left. Then, and only then, are they truly rewarded with the big jobs. The models who stick it out and demand to be noticed eventually *get* noticed if they are good at their jobs, but it really takes passion. Those who don't have it won't last. The agents, the bookers, the producers—all of them participate in this, and it's very harsh because there are always hundreds of girls who will do anything to be models.

I'll never forget when I had the chance to meet with Sephora for a campaign. They were set on booking me, but they wanted to see me first. However, I was in another city at the time and couldn't afford to fly to New York. The agency doesn't pay for the flights or the housing. That's all on the models. I wanted them to book me first, and then I would fly there, knowing I had the job. My agent told me I was blowing a huge opportunity, and there were many, many girls ready to take my place. She even said I was ungrateful, or something like that. I was crying hysterically about it in private, but I stood my ground because it didn't seem fair to make me fly all the way out there just to get looked at when they had all my photos.

This is the kind of thing that prompted me to leave New York and move to Los Angeles. That's when I started writing this book.

One day, I saw this message on my Yogi tea bag: *When ego is lost, limit is lost. You become infinite, beautiful, kind.* Ideally, this is what happens when pride dissolves, but at what cost? I didn't feel I could lose my self-respect or compromise my intelligence just to play that "game," and it *is* a game. Most models have to play it if they want to be really successful, so we all go through this, at least for a while, and some for years. Not me. I had to get out before the whole business started messing with my head.

Eventually, after a year of taking it easy in L.A. and doing less-than-glamorous modeling jobs that actually paid money, I went back to New York. I was more confident, more experienced, and more able to call the shots. Now that I can handle it, I go back and forth, living in New York during the busy seasons, like for Fashion Week, but living primarily in Los Angeles. But it took me a long time to get to the place where I was comfortable doing that. I had to learn how to own my career. But for a while I was seriously over all of that. I realized I had too much self-respect to subject myself to that kind of treatment. I wanted to be a model, but on *my terms*.

Sadly, a lot of girls don't ever get to that point. They stay way too long and submit to way too much before they actually make it! But when they finally do make it, if they make it, I am so relieved for them! Many of the girls at the top now I know personally. I lived with them, I worked with them, and I know how bad it really was! Ironically, I sometimes find myself jealous that they're doing Victoria's Secret or *Sports Illustrated,* but deep down, I know I could be, too—but I wouldn't have this book and the outlook on life that I have. Maybe if I had come from a stronger foundation, a better childhood, I would've been better able to tolerate the way I was treated. But I am who I am. My path has worked out in a way that is right for me and is giving me the platform to do what

I really want to do: help girls and women find the beauty within themselves!

But back to my point: models aren't rich. Most of them barely make it, or they *don't* make it and they have to quit. Many of them live off their parents or their rich boyfriends. Those of us who stick with it do so because we love it, because we're good at it, and because we just happen to have the right kind of look for our clients. Sure, some models also go into it for the attention—maybe the attention they didn't get as kids. But it's definitely not about the money.

■ ■

So there you have it—the "skinny" on what it's really like to be a model. It can be harsh, and it can be fun. It can be enlightening, and it can be tedious. It's like any other job. And, like any other job, we are specialists at what we do, and what we do is *look good,* despite our imperfections, oddities, and weaknesses.

That means most models know some things that other people might not know, especially if their appearance isn't the major influencing factor governing their income. We have secrets. We have strategies. We have *modeltude.* (This is also in the Urban Dictionary!)

FashionSpeak

Modeltude is my term for the way models project themselves to the world. It includes a lot: the way models carry themselves; their posture; their state of mind or disposition; and their general attitude toward life, food, sex, beauty, and weight. To have modeltude means to keep your head up, shoulders back, chest out, and core in. It also means moving through life looking and feeling like a supermodel—not arrogant, vain, or brainless, but strong, beautiful, confident, and powerful.

And that brings me straight into the main point of this book: How do we do it? Are you ready to learn the secrets, too?

■ ■ ■

CHAPTER THREE

The Supermodel YOU Secret Formula

As for diets . . . anything with the word <u>die</u> in it you probably want to avoid! I'd say eat what gives you the motivation and energy to be active. That keeps you confident and teaches you discipline and consistency. I run around the city all day for castings, so I find healthy snacking several times a day keeps my tank running. Modeling is something that takes a lot of strength and persistence, and if we eat right and stay clear of negative energy, we can dominate this business.

— ERIN AXTELL, SUPER-REAL AND SUPERBEAUTIFUL MODEL, REPRESENTED BY NEXT MODELS, NEW YORK

I'm guessing you picked up this book for one primary reason. Maybe you're curious about the lives of models, but I'll bet what you want to know most (since it's the question I get *asked* the most, by far) is: "How do models stay so skinny?"

You want that for yourself. You want a supermodel body. I get it! And I want to help you get the body you want. I also want you to glow with self-confidence. I want you to feel sexy and adorable. I want your posture to reflect how much you love yourself. I want you to radiate beauty. I want you to channel your inner supermodel—the very best, most gorgeous, most elegant, most aesthetically pleasing *you,* inside and out.

So I'm going to share the model secret formula for getting your supermodel body. It's not complicated, yet not every model could exactly articulate it because it just comes naturally to us. We live it. *You* can live it, too. This is what everything in this book is helping you to achieve, and it's really pretty simple.

Remember, our genes do not determine how much weight we carry. They influence overall body shape or type, but not weight. More than 90 percent of my family members are overweight, but I'm not, and you don't have to be, either, no matter what your mother or sisters look like. *You are not destined to be overweight.*

The real reason healthy models stay *skealthy* isn't that they go on diets, kill themselves at the gym, or deny themselves the pleasure of their favorite foods. It's just this: they are in energy balance.

What Is Energy Balance?

There's a reason why models learn how to walk with books on their heads. (I never actually did this, but when I was little, I remember thinking that's what models were supposed to do!) They're learning balance. Physical balance. But models also have to learn energy balance if they are going to keep the bodies that get them the jobs. You can learn energy balance, too, and it's crucial to understand if you really want to channel your inner supermodel.

Energy balance is a simple concept: it is the situation in which you take in as much energy as you burn. You are in energy balance when your energy intake (food and beverages) balances or equals your energy output from your resting metabolic rate, or RMR (which is your internal heat, or how much energy you expend just sitting on your cute butt), and external work (exercise, movement, shopping, dancing, and so forth). When this equation works, you are in energy balance.

You can even write it like a math equation, if you're into that kind of thing:

Energy Balance Formula

Energy Intake (EI) = Resting Metabolic Rate (RMR) + External Work (EW)

or

EI = RMR + EW

Too math-geeky? I totally agree (and I consider myself a *smart model!*). So, to put it more simply, energy balance just means eating an amount of food that is equivalent to the amount of energy your body personally requires. Not much more, and definitely no less. This is the secret most models have mastered without always being totally aware of it. They can just feel how much their bodies need. We are all born knowing this. Babies are born knowing how much milk they need. Children know how much they want to eat, but the more we are subjected to the modern world, the more we forget. The point is to re-member it, or better yet, to never forget it. Models have reclaimed this ability. Some of them learn it by counting calories, or figuring out how many calories are in their favorite foods, and estimating how much they burn just going about their day. This is a technical approach that can help you learn how to once again feel when you are truly full. Oth-ers don't get so technical, but they are so self-aware that they can tell when they've had too much. They tune in to their cravings and their satisfaction level while eating, and they know exactly when to stop. It's an art, it's a science—and for models, it's a necessity.

It would be nice if I could just tell you exactly how many calories you should eat and let you go off counting them, but the body is more complex than that. The amount of food you need to eat will change as you gain or lose weight. It will increase or decrease as your metabolism and physical activity change. But no matter how the numbers shift, both sides of the equation have to balance. Imagine standing on a teeter-totter, trying to keep it level to the ground. It's tricky, but once you get the hang of it, it's a lot easier than it was at first.

But energy balance is only relevant once you've reached the weight you want to be. If you are trying to lose weight, you've got to shift the teeter-totter a bit to one side—you've got to use slightly more energy than you take in. This is difficult because of homeostasis. *Homeostasis* is the equilibrium your body finds at whatever weight you've been for an extended period of time. Even if you're under- or overweight, if you maintain a steady weight for a certain amount of time, your body will acclimate to that set point by adjusting its own metabolism, and then it will try to stay there, at that equilibrium it has achieved. Our bodies are amazing machines in this way.

In our early evolution, this was superhelpful for survival. Gaining weight was a good thing because it was a protection against future food shortages, so our bodies are hardwired to make weight gain easy and weight loss difficult. Because what if a famine hits? What if you are starving? Somebody should tell our bodies it's the 21st century!

But until someone figures out how to deliver that message, we need to deal with homeostasis—and not just deal with it, but make it work *for* us. When you weigh more or less than is right for your body, you might be in homeostasis, but it's going to be a shakier homeostasis, like trying to keep that teeter-totter balanced with one side at a 45-degree angle. *Way* harder than keeping it level! It's possible, but it kind of sucks.

So you need to get your body back to the place where the balance feels the best—that horizontal teeter-totter, that Supermodel YOU place you want to be.

The most important way to do this is to balance the Five Keys, which I'll talk about in the next five chapters. But for now, let's talk about what you can do to help tweak your body back into a healthy and stable energy balance right now.

Let's begin by imagining you just lying on the couch. No judgment—I love to lie on the couch! But let's consider what you need while you're lying there, channel surfing or listening to your new playlist or just taking a little catnap.

You need energy to breathe. You need energy for your heart to pump. You need energy for your blood to circulate through your body, to eliminate waste products, and for all that brain activity, even if it's just sweet dreams about the body or job or hottie of your dreams. That energy has to come from somewhere.

Now imagine that you get up from the couch and go for a walk or a run, or you go dancing or shopping, or you clean your bathroom. You're going to need even more energy now because of all the muscles you're using. How much more depends on your individual body composition and size. For example, a 125-pound model and a 225-pound football player are going to expend totally different amounts of energy walking one block, let alone dancing at a club.

Eat to Burn

The way your metabolism alone works in your individual body to use energy is mind-boggling, at least to a model like me! You could never actually calculate the number of calories to equal your inner burn because it's based on moment-to-moment changes in your biochemistry, your unique build, what kind of food you've recently eaten, and the way you use your body.

However, you can make a pretty good estimate—good enough to start moving your body into a more desirable homeostatic state. Start with your resting metabolic rate, or RMR. It's the bare minimum number of calories you need in order to exist—basically, lying on that couch. If you plan to use more energy, you need more calories, so if you move more, you need to eat more. But if you dip below this rate, that's when the chaos starts. You'll start storing fat because your body thinks it's in famine mode. You'll be tired and have no energy, because that's exactly what calories are: energy! Go without enough calories for too long, get obsessive about it, and you could even become anorexic.

Nerd Alert!

Your RMR is important, but I don't want you to think of it as a maximum. Remember, it's a minimum. You can't go under it, but you can go over it. Actually, the more you eat, the more you burn. I recently read this study that showed that female gymnasts and runners who didn't eat for three hours or longer had the highest body-fat percentages compared to those who snacked more often, even if they weren't consuming more calories than they were burning. The longer the gap between meals or snacks, the higher the level of body fat, especially when they exercised during those non-eating periods.

So it's not even remotely as simple as burning as many calories at the gym as you eat in your diet. You aren't a math formula. You're a beautiful, complex, miraculous being who defies and exceeds any mere formula. But if you do want to lose weight, you need to shift your balance gradually to a new set point, a new balance point: your ideal weight point.

Here's a good formula to help you figure this out. Now don't get all freaked out by the math equation. It's easy, and you know your cell phone has a calculator, so you can take 30 seconds to do these simple calculations. This is the formula for women (men end up being able to have more calories because they generally have more muscle mass, so they burn calories faster—so unfair, right?). Before doing the calculation, convert your weight to kilograms by taking your weight in pounds and multiplying by 0.45. Use that number in the formula below:

RMR Formula

(10 × weight in kilograms) + (6.25 × height in inches) + (5 × age) – 161 = RMR

Now, multiply your RMR by the number that represents your activity level:

Activity Level Number

1.2—You're pretty lazy, don't exercise, always drive, etc. You are like most girls—at least, most models.

1.375—You do light exercise one to three days a week, like walking the dog, taking the stairs, etc. You try . . . a little.

1.55—You do moderate exercise or sports three to five days a week. You're a rock star!

1.725—You're very active and do hard exercise or sports six to seven days a week. You're the girl version of Rambo!

1.9—You're extremely active and do hard daily exercise or sports and have a physical job. You're my hero! Do you mind if I sit on the couch and admire you?

Your RMR × your Activity Level Number = the *minimum* number of calories you need to eat every day to maintain your weight.

Now, if you want to *lose* weight, just do this same formula, but plug in the weight number you're going for. That will give you the minimum number of calories to start changing your shape.

A lot of models never count calories. I actually do. I love being aware of exactly what I'm eating, and keeping track like this helps my awareness. I also keep track of about how many calories I burn when I do any kind of exercise, like yoga or spin class. Since I'm vegan, I want to be extra-sure that I'm getting enough protein for pretty hair and nails, and enough fat for beautiful skin. I also like knowing that I'm getting all of my nutrients or not OD'ing on green juice or carrots or whatever it may be!

MODEL **TALK**

It looks as though we have hit a new generation of models. Now, instead of not eating or throwing up everything, they have become health nuts!

— Adria Ali, supertrainer (**www.fittipdaily.com**)

Some pretty good apps for phones and computers will help you track this stuff, and I recommend finding one you like (check out Appendix B for suggestions). Knowing about how many calories you need, how many calories you're eating, how many calories you're burning, and what nutrients are in the food you eat helps a lot with self-awareness (the first key, which I'll talk about in the next chapter), especially if you tend to be oblivious about what you're putting in your mouth. If you know, then you can guesstimate your activity level, and it helps you have an idea about your body's needs.

The beauty of the energy-balance method is that you never have to worry about what you're supposed to eat or stick to some plan you hate or whatever. Yawn! Models have their favorite foods, and nobody is going to tell them they can't have them! Instead, we just stay in balance, and our bodies stay *super!*

I've also noticed a trend in the modeling world: we tend to choose natural, whole, and nutrient-dense foods made from the earth and not in a lab. This lets us stay in energy balance while *getting to eat more.* This is one of the biggest reasons why models stay so thin but still eat so much. We learn to love, and thrive on, foods that nourish us, as opposed to junk like fast food and sugar that has zero benefits or links to improving our looks. This is why models eat healthier—we eat in a way that makes us look and feel better, and gives us that all-important energy we need to spend hours modeling clothes, doing quick changes, or enduring marathon hair and makeup sessions.

It sounds simple, but it can take a while to master. I do it naturally now—I just know what I need to eat to stay in energy balance. You might not know today, but with some calculations and label-reading, and by keeping track of a few things on your smartphone or a good old-fashioned piece of paper, you'll get it, and then it will become a habit.

MODEL **TALK**

Those old habits don't have to be erased; they just become replaced by a new habit that is more in vibrational harmony with who you are and what you want.

—Abraham, via Esther and Jerry Hicks, super–spiritual life-changers

What Are You Eating?

Another essential part of staying in energy balance is choosing foods that will maintain your energy and make you look prettier. It helps to know a few things, like how antioxidants (in brightly colored fruits and vegetables, and yummy drinks like green tea) and omega-3 fatty acids (in nuts, seeds, and fish) give you gorgeous skin; how protein gives you energy and strength; and how fiber keeps your tummy flat. It's also important to eat the foods that make you feel good. For me, that's vegan, raw food, but for some people, that's a lot of fish or lean meat, no grains, or whatever works for them.

Just like you can't be or look like someone else or have someone else's body, you also can't assume that someone else's dietary choices will be right for you. And the only way to really know what foods make you feel like Supermodel YOU is to cultivate your self-awareness. Not only can you learn to feel when you are in energy balance, but you can also learn which foods make you feel energetic versus tired, bloated versus sleek, radiant versus dull, rosy versus pale, or animated versus sluggish. Pay attention! Your food choices matter, and they shouldn't have anything to do with some diet plan (unless you like to follow those—some people love to have someone just tell them exactly what to eat). It should be all about how you look and feel eating in a particular way.

Modeltude

Are you a label whore? Let's face it, many of us would love a Louis Vuitton bag or two, and a closet full of Christian Louboutins and Manolo Blahniks, but most models don't have the money to afford the things they wear on the runway. But that doesn't mean you have to dress like a frump. Go into H&M, Forever 21, and vintage stores. Models are notoriously good at spotting the great finds at the cheapest prices. Buy the clothes, shoes, and handbags you can afford so you don't stress out about money. If it looks good and feels good, who cares if it came from Target?

But there *is* a time to be a label whore: when it comes to food! Read the ingredient labels. Be a total snob about it. Less is more, and unpronounceable ingredients are a big food-fashion faux pas. Don't worry about calories or fat—you need those! The higher the protein, usually the better for energy. Sugar is a bad idea. I always check the sugar first—I hate that stuff! Sugar is bad for your body and definitely bad for your face, accelerating aging inside and out. Especially avoid high-fructose corn syrup! Many studies in both children and adults suggest that it is a major contributor to the obesity epidemic.

If you feel good, you'll look good. And there is no better way to feel good than to be a total snob about what you put into (rather than onto) your body.

It's time to wake up to your choices. Think about the first time you ever tried soda. Did your eyes water? Did it sting your throat? What about beer? Did you get that bitter beer face? When you first tried a cigarette, did you practically cough up a lung or feel like your throat was on fire for the next 24 hours? But the more you kept drinking or smoking these things, the more you ignored the signs from your body and the fainter those signals became—until your body just stopped sending them.

This kind of body intuition is something you have to relearn, but you were born knowing it, so you can reclaim it! It isn't necessarily easy at first, if you aren't used to doing it, but keep reminding yourself that you have the inner knowledge. If it's difficult for you, just start practicing. The best way to start is to learn the Five Keys to channeling your inner supermodel.

Introducing the Five Keys

After reading a ton of really smart, really boring research and initiating top-secret observation of (*read:* spying on) my fellow models, what I discovered is that there are basically five key elements that affect body weight, health, vitality, and beauty, and they are the same for all of us.

I call these the *Five Keys to Channeling Your Inner Supermodel,* but what I mean by that is the *Five Keys to Energy Balance.* These are not only the keys to your dream body, but also the keys to health, happiness, and ultimately your dream life. You need all five, because they work together. Like a model and her iPhone, you cannot separate them! And once you have them down, your health habits will run on autopilot. You won't even have to think about them anymore.

Most of the healthy models I know have these keys mastered without even necessarily realizing it. These are not difficult concepts to understand (thank goodness, for me and models everywhere, who are too fidgety to sit down and listen to difficult concepts for very long!). But they are vital to finding your inner supermodel and achieving a supermodel body.

Practicing all of these keys together will help you achieve *your* dream body and dream life. I'll go into detail in upcoming chapters, but here's a preview of how easy this can all be, so you can start thinking and acting like a supermodel *right now.*

There is a very good reason why self-awareness is the first key. You can't accomplish any of the other keys effectively without it. You'll just rationalize away all your bad health habits. Without self-awareness, it's too easy to blame other factors, other people, fate, or whatever you can think of to avoid responsibility for your own happiness.

When you live with self-awareness, you will know when you're really hungry and when you're just bored or nervous or sad. You will notice when you're full, instead of eating way past that point. You'll feel when you need to move more, and you'll feel when it's time to rest. You'll know when you need sleep, and you'll know why you need it. It all begins here. I'll tell you more about self-awareness and how to achieve it in the next chapter.

Being a model can be pretty harsh sometimes. The industry is completely unpredictable. As Heidi Klum famously states on *Project Runway,* "In fashion, one day you are in, and the next you are out." It's the same with all aspects of fashion, including modeling. Your look or body can be revered one day and passé the next. You can be in demand, then nobody wants to hire you anymore, with no warning. So as a model, you pretty much never know what to expect. You have to be prepared for anything, and that's stressful. This is one of the reasons why the Five Keys I'm going to talk about in the next section are so crucial for survival, not to mention health and beauty.

If you neglect any one of the Five Keys, you are likely to experience signs that your body is out of balance. These are like signal flares sent up to get your attention. They can be anything in your body that you don't like, or that you know isn't good, from weight gain to insomnia; bad skin to constant fatigue; low energy to that jacked-up, disaster-impending feeling you get when you've been under too much stress for too long. Do you experience any of these signs of imbalance?

Take these as a warning that you need to change something. I do this all the time. Every time I have any discomfort, I ask myself why. My stomach hurts. *Why?* I'm grumpy. *Why?* I just ate garbage. *Why?* I don't have any energy. *Why?* These are all signs that your equation isn't working, and amazing opportunities for you to figure out *why,* so you can get back into balance.

KEY 1:
Self-Awareness

Self-awareness is the premier key. It is the most important, the *número uno,* and without it, none of the other keys will work. It's central to everything in your life, not just losing weight. Truly *everything.*

Being self-aware means understanding the reasons behind what you do: why you choose to eat the food you eat, how it makes you feel after you eat it, how you sleep, how you move . . . everything. It means consciously perceiving your body's experience in the world and *not* running on autopilot all day long. It means paying attention to yourself, your body, your mind, and what's going on around you.

For example, self-awareness means that before I make a food choice or decide whether to go out or do anything else, I am aware that I have an early-morning flight the next day. I know I will need eight hours of sleep to be functional and healthy, so I plan my afternoon and evening to make sure I get what I need. I also know I'll need to pack the night before, and get mentally prepared for the trip. Self-awareness means I know that I should pack snacks, just in case I get stranded without any food. It means checking the weather, picking out appropriate clothes, and eating a balanced dinner so I can get the sleep I need. Eating the right foods helps you sleep, especially if the foods contain healthy fats. Eating sugar at night, however, can interfere with sleep. And don't eat right before bed! Going to bed on a full stomach means digesting all night long instead of repairing cells for morning beauty!

For me, self-awareness also means breathing deeply and maybe meditating so I'm less nervous on the flight. I used to be a wreck before I boarded a plane, nervous about both flying and the assignment ahead, but now that I've become more self-aware, I have the process down. Sometimes I still worry that I haven't packed everything I need, but I've also learned that there is a point when I just have to let it all go. I will never be 100 percent ready or have everything I might need, but as long as I have the essentials, I'll be fine. Accepting this is part of self-awareness, too—so much so that travel is actually relaxing to me now, and the only time I get to catch up on movies!

Self-awareness is part of all of this. It means a million other things I couldn't even list—conscious and subconscious actions that all align to get me where I need to be, in the state of being required for the job. It means integrating and practicing good habits so I stay in balance. Good habits are a huge part of the reason why healthy models can master these keys. When features like our posture and how our hands look in photos become habits, we don't have to force them. Models have this key down. Body language becomes a product of self-awareness, rather than something random or subconscious. But even if your profession has nothing to do with your body, you are living your whole *life* in that body of yours, so you owe it to yourself to use it correctly and with conscious intention, rather than blundering through life without paying attention to the vehicle for your spirit! C'mon. This is important! Especially considering that being unhappy with one's body is the number one reported cause of unhappiness in women and girls.

It's time to let go of any excuses for why you don't have the body of your dreams, and start paying attention to *why* you don't have the body of your dreams. Excuses diminish your power and your purpose. You are not a victim. You are powerful beyond your wildest dreams. All you have to do is pay attention.

MODEL **TALK**

Our deepest fear is not that we are inadequate. Our deepest fear is that we are powerful beyond measure. It is our light, not our darkness, that most frightens us. We ask ourselves, "Who am I to be brilliant, gorgeous, talented, fabulous?" Actually, who are you not to be? You are a child of God. Your playing small does not serve the world. There is nothing enlightened about shrinking so that other people won't feel insecure around you. We are all meant to shine, as children do. We were born to make manifest the glory of God that is within us. It's not just in some of us; it's in everyone. And as we let our own light shine, we unconsciously give other people permission to do the same. As we are liberated from our own fear, our presence automatically liberates others.

— Marianne Williamson, superauthor and spiritual activist
(from *A Return to Love*)

KEY 2:
Beauty Sleep

I love to sleep. Sleep is awesome . . . when you can get it. But we often don't get enough. In fact, for most of us, a good night's rest is something that only happens once in a while, and that's too bad because beauty sleep is Key 2, and it's absolutely essential for functioning at your peak and having the body of your dreams.

I totally understand the predicament. I have a hard time getting a good night's sleep, and I'm such a light sleeper that I wake up at the slightest noise. And I know what it's like to be really busy. But if your rockin' nightlife, schoolwork, or family life takes precedence over rest, you're going to pay a price.

Models make beauty sleep a priority because we know it affects our appearance, mind, and appetite, and when any of these things get out of balance, our work will suffer. A lot of models I know might not necessarily think very far beyond *If I don't sleep, I'm going to look terrible tomorrow!* But the end result is that models sleep like they are getting paid for it, and in some ways, they are.

Looking good and getting paid depend on each other, and models have to pay the rent, too.

But good, sound sleep won't come without self-awareness, so this key builds on the last one. In Chapter 5, I'll tell you how to get the seven to eight hours of snoozing we all need, but usually don't get.

MODEL **TALK**

Sixty-four percent of Americans get less than eight hours of sleep per night, while 32 percent get less than six. That's a lot of tired people!

— Dr. Michael Breus, superpsychologist and sleep doctor
(via Twitter: @thesleepdoctor)

KEY 3:
De-stressing

No one purposely seeks out stress, but it's part of daily life, and if you don't know how to deal with it, you're going to get out of balance. Models are typically under a lot of stress, just as I'm sure you are. They have crazy work schedules, inconsistent and unstable pay, big bills . . . OMG, I'm getting stressed just thinking about it all!

We know that stress can lead to overeating and packing on extra pounds, but models have to pack bags, not pounds—they can't afford that kind of extra baggage! So we absolutely have to know how to deal with stress. But again, without self-awareness—and in addition, without adequate sleep—you may not even realize you're stressed. And that stress can wreck all your good intentions and foil all your established good habits. And then you fall apart.

I would guess that a model's number one stressor is money. Maybe it's your number one stressor, too. Yep, that cold, hard cash can really do a number on us. At least we're not alone. According to the American Psychological Association, money is the number one cause of stress in America. But there are plenty of other stressors to choose from, and you might not even realize some of the things that are causing you stress because you're just so used to it that you now mistake "stressed" for "how I normally feel."

MODEL **PLAYLIST**

I play gospel in the morning because I like to start my day feeling blessed, and thinking and feeling positive and ready for the day. Then I like listening to slow R&B, like Floetry or Erykah Badu, just to stay relaxed, because the day can get pretty crazy and overwhelming.

— Eugena Washington, second runner-up on *America's Next Top Model,* represented by Major Model Management New York

---

When I was in full show circuit—that means doing the shows in all the major fashion cities—and I was working wild hours and flying constantly to New York, Milan, and Paris, my face broke out 24/7. I blamed it on the makeup, which didn't help, but that wasn't the cause. It was *stress* that jacked up my hormones, made it impossible for me to *sleep,* and made me break out. Period.

And speaking of periods, being so freakin' stressed can stop your period, too, which also happened to me. It wasn't my diet or an eating disorder. It was stress that made me put the tampons back on the shelf.

Now, I'm not totally oblivious. I know that some models, like a minority of people in any profession, deal with stress in unhealthy ways. Some might smoke or drink or do something even worse for the body, mind, and spirit, but for skealthy models who don't go there, it's crucial to figure out health-boosting, supermodel-body stress-management techniques.

In Chapter 6, I'll share all the model secrets I know for keeping stress at bay, like music for chilling out and meditation methods that actually work. It's true! Meditation isn't what you might imagine. I think people associate meditation with the vision of monks in Tibet—legs crossed, eyes closed, chanting "Om" or some other weird thing—but it doesn't have to be anything like that. Meditation is essentially quieting your mind and focusing inward, and it's a major stress reliever! Many models do this by simply popping in their earphones and detaching from the craziness or negativity around them.

Model Behavior

Even if all of this energy-balance business makes perfect sense to you, you may still have trouble following through, and that's another issue, although it's related to balance. It's about motivation.

This is important, so pay attention: One of the reasons why models are thin is because they have to be. As I've said, it's part of the job. This is a huge motivator for a model, so we can't overlook this. In your job, you might have to be really good at something—like studying, public speaking, writing, using computers, teaching, or cooking—but gaining weight doesn't really matter that much for getting your paycheck.

To a model, it's everything. Gaining weight is not an option! So if you really want a supermodel body, you're going to have to start thinking this way. You need to decide that being overweight is simply not an option for you. Being skealthy is now part of your job description, whatever you do. You have no alternative but to inhabit your dream body. Achieving your ideal weight is *required.* You will reach your natural perfect weight and love your body, and that's just the way it is.

Models are seriously committed to their bodies, and you can be committed to yours, too. After all, having the body of your dreams will make you happier, because you will feel better, healthier, and more beautiful. (I'll talk more about this in Chapter 8.)

KEY 4:
Modercizing

Forget exercise. It's so boring and time-consuming. Models hardly ever do it. But they do modercize, and that's plenty.

FashionSpeak

Modercize is the model version of exercise, and it just means movement. It's natural movement that's part of your real life, not some artificial movement you do just for the sake of exercise.

Movement counts as exercise! Models get a lot of exercise, but they do it in the context of their lives, not hidden away in a gym somewhere lifting weights for no reason or running for miles just to get back to where they started. Those are modern-day replacements for all the physical work our ancestors would get every day as they lived their lives just trying to find food and survive. It's true that these days, a lot of people just sit all day at computers, but there are better, more natural, more fun, less boring ways to get your butt in gear than by going to the gym.

Models burn calories by walking on the beach (or playing beach volleyball, if somebody suggests it—who doesn't love a sport you can play in a bikini?), working (all that runway work and changing clothes over and over is more strenuous than it looks), dancing (anybody wanna go clubbing?), shopping (bargain hunting—and I mean the getting-out-and-walking-around kind, not the browsing-on-eBay kind), and fidgeting. Models are notoriously fidgety, and that adds up to tons of calories burned—just by tapping your foot or shifting back and forth. Even vacuuming counts. And washing dishes.

Remember that study I told you about in the last chapter, where the cleaning ladies who knew they were burning calories lost weight, while the ones who didn't know didn't change at all? Modercizing is just living an active life, but *knowing* you are doing so. Again, this goes back to self-awareness. Move, notice that you're moving, and it counts! With self-awareness, adequate sleep, and a good diet, modercizing will have the ultimate effect. Try it! Get up and do something. And notice your body when you do it. It's easy, it's natural, and when you get in the habit of just moving more while you're doing whatever you're doing anyway, you'll be exercising the way models do it.

I'll tell you a lot more about how to do this in Chapter 7. Meanwhile, are you tapping your foot right now? Maybe fidgeting just a little? And are you feeling even prettier, thinner, and more confident as you read this? Yes, you are!

MODEL **TALK**

So many people can't find the time to exercise, but any little movement is better than sitting still. In fact, fidgeting can burn up to 300 calories. So, tap your fingers, wiggle your toes, move your hips.

— Dr. Mehmet Oz, America's favorite superdoctor

KEY 5:
Intuitive Eating

I've already established that models eat. We don't starve ourselves. We eat. But the *way* to stay skinny is the real secret of Key 5. Here is what skealthy models know: dieting makes you fat. For real. But skealthy-model intuitive-eating techniques will have just the opposite effect.

Intuitive eating is what children do. They eat when they're hungry, and they eat as much as they need because they aren't yet swayed by junk food and weird societal eating patterns and habits. Intuitive eating helps you reclaim your natural intuition about what you need to eat, and how much you need to eat, to stay in energy balance.

Intuitive eating is a way of eating that taps directly into Key 1, self-awareness. When you are fully aware of your body, you notice how you feel when you eat certain things, and when you don't like the results, you realize you don't want to eat those things anymore. This is an art and it takes a while to master, but your body is the ultimate authority on the food you need. Once you break through the bad habits and mindless eating, you'll discover a whole new way that is uniquely yours and uniquely suited to giving you the body of your dreams.

But as you can probably already see, without self-awareness, adequate sleep, and stress management, it's going to be a lot more difficult to get control of your eating. You have to be practicing the first three keys if you want the power to master this one. And if you want to eat more? Then move more! That's what models do. Many of them say that they increase exercise on the days when they want to indulge more.

Models have learned all of this as a matter of career survival, but we also have a few other tricks up our fashionable sleeves. I'll talk about more of them in Chapter 8, but let me give you just a few teasers. These are some of my favorite intuitive-eating techniques:

— **Eat pretty.** If you think about how you look when you eat, you might just change your style. You can even watch yourself eat in a mirror. Is it cringe-worthy, or is it pretty? Taking small bites is pretty. Chewing with your mouth closed is pretty. Not making noise when you eat is pretty. Do those three things and you'll consume about 20 percent less than the chick chomping away at the next table.

— **Think small.** Use small plates and serve yourself small portions. Then check in: How do you feel? If you really want more, have more. Or maybe you need less than you thought. I always use these tiny bowls and spoons, and people laugh at me, but it really does help me keep portions under control and not eat more than my body really wants or needs.

— **Write it down.** Write down what you eat, and also how you feel before and after. You can keep a food journal, or keep track on your phone or computer or any way you want, but do it. It's the quickest way to self-awareness about what you eat and how it affects you. This isn't about making you feel guilty or forcing portion control. It's about training your self-awareness so you're more likely to remember how gross you felt the last time you ate a hot dog or a whole pint of ice cream. This is important! I used to always have terrible stomachaches and gas. How unsexy is that? It was because I wasn't digesting the food I was eating. My body was trying to tell me, *Hey! I don't like this! Stop feeding me this!* But it wasn't until I started writing down what I was eating that I finally made the connection between particular foods and my body's re-action to them. Finally, I was able to start listening. Excessive gas and constipation are not natural. They are signals. Pay attention by writing down what you eat and how your body responds, and you'll figure it out. If you keep letting 'em rip or you can't poo, no-tice it! Self-awareness meets intuitive eating through journaling!

In Appendix A, I'll also give you some daily menus and favor-ite foods from real models so you can see what we tend to eat. No, it's not just baby carrots! You'll see that some models eat meat; some eat candy; some eat pasta; and many of them eat delicious exotic dishes from their home countries, like Norwegian fish balls or Brazilian barbecue or the Russian dumplings called *pelmeni*.

Models are notorious snackers, too, and we often eat dessert, including chocolate, sugar, or whatever we want. The trick is not overdoing it—self-awareness keeps you in check, and pigging out is not pretty. Eating what you want while listening to your body will keep you in energy balance. It's crazy diets and skipping meals that throw you out of whack.

So that's the big secret: the fancy-schmancy equation that will keep you in energy balance, and the Five Keys that will help you achieve it. You need all five in order to be Supermodel YOU be-cause they depend on each other, but they're easy, they're fun, and I'm going to walk you through all of them, step-by-step, in the next five chapters.

Let's get fired up with modeltude—remember, that's a state of mind, a disposition, the way you carry yourself, and the way you let your inner supermodel shine. So strike a pose! We're going to get with the Supermodel YOU program.

And in the meantime, if it makes you feel even more balanced, you can practice walking in four-inch stilettos with a book on your head.

■ ■ ■

CHAPTER FOUR

Key 1: Self-Awareness

Awareness is the first step in healing or changing.

— LOUISE HAY, ONE OF THE WORLD'S BIGGEST SUPER (ROLE) MODELS

How self-aware do you think you are? I mean this literally. Do you think you really know yourself? Do you think you are eating that cupcake or that candy bar because you're genuinely hungry? Do you think you are sitting all crooked like that in your chair because it's more comfortable and better for your body? Do you think you are wearing the clothes you really want to wear? Are you comfortable? Do you feel good? Do you even notice how you feel?

Do you think you walk into a room in a way that makes you seem invisible or insecure? Do you think you can't live without sugar? Do you think you are squinting or straining your eyes when you read this? Do you think you are smiling? Do you think you are breathing deeply? Do you think you are focusing on what you really should be focusing on right now? Do you think you are tired or bored or anxious or peaceful? Do you think you are acting like yourself, or do you feel like something's "off"?

Do you think you are self-aware?

Self-awareness is where all change begins. That's why it is the first key. Without self-awareness, you'll never have the ability to understand why you are where you are or what you need to do to change anything, be it your body, your energy, your health, or your life. By developing self-awareness, you'll be able to self-actualize all your desires. Otherwise, forget it. You're just going to be swept along by fate, with no say in where you end up.

Although you might not have guessed this before reading this book, models actually have a high level of self-awareness. We have to be self-aware because it's part of our job to know how we look, how we photograph, how we stand, and how we walk. We can't go all Hunchback-of-Notre-Dame down the runway. We have to know exactly how our faces look when we make different expressions, and how clothes look on us when we stand one way as opposed to another way. We constantly have to be aware of our posture and the messages we are sending with our body language. These are all important aspects of being a good model.

SUPERMODEL **SAYS . . .**

Dig deep within yourself to find your true self and let that guide you through life.

— Fatma Dabo, super-regal Gambian model

Let me give you an example of how important this is.

One of the first jobs I did with Versace was for an event in their store on Rodeo Drive. They had hired three models, and our job was to be mannequins, standing on top of pillars, decked out head to toe in Versace. Stacie, the head of Versace PR, informed us that we had to stay as still as possible, just like real mannequins, moving only to change our position if we absolutely needed to. We were not allowed to talk to the guests, smile, or respond in any way. She also warned us to be careful because a girl in New York had actually passed out and fallen off the pillar doing a job just like this one. Who knew modeling was so dangerous? (Actually, I could tell you stories—falling off a horse while shooting in Cannes, hanging out of the back of a moving U-Haul truck for a shoot, climbing a barbed-wire fence in Paris, discovering leeches in the water that caused me to freak out and splash water all over the expensive camera equipment—ah yes, my glamorous life!)

You have no idea how incredibly hard this is! I dare you to put on the most ridiculously high and uncomfortable heels you can find, strike a mannequin-like pose, and hold it for even five minutes. The two other girls and I had to do this for much longer! We would hold a pose for 25 to 30 minutes, go change our clothes, and then go back and do it again.

This is what happens when you have to stay still in extreme positions for an extended period of time: Your leg starts to fall asleep, or your arm, or multiple limbs at once. You start to shake, your hip starts to give, you get crazy itches you can't scratch. On top of the physical challenge, you've got all of these people staring at you and poking you and wondering if you're real, or freaking out when they realize you are. Or they're trying to get you to break face.

This was the most challenging job I've probably ever done as a model, and I'm telling you about it because it was an amazing exercise in self-awareness. I had to gain complete control over my body and mind. It was a total-body workout and a meditation all in one. I felt like I consciously experienced every muscle in my body and became keenly aware of my breath, my heartbeat, and what every part of me was doing, from scalp to fingers to the bottoms of my feet.

And I was good at it! People thought I was a real mannequin. The other models had a harder time. One of the girls had to get down before we were finished, and the third girl kept moving or laughing when people would try to break her. Not me. Once they realized I was real, people at the event kept trying to get me to laugh. Eventually, they succeeded when an NBA player kept offering me a drink of his champagne, and then put his glass to my lips and started to pour his drink into my mouth. I couldn't help laughing, but I credit my ability to do the job so well (at least up to that point) to self-awareness.

That lesson stayed with me. I started to notice things in my everyday life, like the fact that I tend to rest more weight on my right hip when I'm standing or washing the dishes or brushing my teeth. I also noticed that I didn't always distribute my weight properly while walking or standing, which tired me out faster. I always wore out the outer edges of my shoes first—no wonder I was prone to turning my ankle! No wonder my high school basketball coach had to tape up my ankles before every game! Think about your life and look for clues like this that will tell you how you use your body. Are you slouching or leaning, standing, or sitting crooked? How is your posture? Posture is so important for models because it can totally change how you look and the energy you project. When you distribute your body weight properly, roll your shoulders back, hold your head up, and tighten your core muscles, you'll almost always feel more energetic. You'll feel better, and you'll look thinner and prettier.

Most people don't notice how they distribute their weight, how long their strides are, how well they stay balanced, or how they stand or sit. Paying attention to your posture is the very first step in Key 1: self-awareness. When you learn to notice and then to control your weight distribution, and you carry yourself with pride and confidence—upright and tall, with a tight core and chest forward—you will burn more calories and turn more heads. And all of that leads to greater sensitivity to and self-awareness about what's going on in your brain, from the thoughts that run through your head all day to the words you choose to say (helpful or hurtful?), to the decisions you make about what to eat, what to focus on, what to love.

What do models know about self-awareness? A lot. Here's why. . . .

The Self-Conscious Model

Self-awareness and its dark side, self-consciousness, are particular issues for models because we are constantly criticized and judged, but also praised and held up on a pedestal. It can be very confusing for some models, especially the youngest ones, but it can also be illuminating for the models who can learn to take in the information and use it.

Here's the tricky part: Models are treated in a very inconsistent manner by everyone, from the industry to the public. On one hand, everybody treats models like they are somehow superior. For example, when people find out I'm a model, many say that they wish *they* could be a model or have always wanted to be one. But on the other hand, often in the same breath, people insult us—they make cracks about our health or probable drug addiction, our bodies, our attitudes, and especially our intelligence. Talk about mixed messages!

The industry is probably the hardest on us, as I've already explained. We are criticized for our posture; how we walk; what we wear; our hair, nails, teeth, and skin; and even how we smell! I'm totally serious! I can't tell you how many times models are told not to wear perfume to a job or are accused of showing up with BO, and maybe that's not professional, but the people we work with have no problem cutting down models who have committed something they perceive as a transgression. Excuse *us!* As an example, these are some of the e-mails my agent sends out to us before jobs. They aren't exactly subtle:

- Arrive hair- and makeup-ready. Nobody has time to sit around and wait for you. Do it on your own time.

- Nude bra and G-string only. Don't be an idiot. Pink, orange, etc., do not count as nude!

- Arrive with a nude mani/pedi. Again, *nude means nude!* Don't waste everybody's time having your nails done at the job, and don't be like the girl who recently arrived at a job with neon-green nails. You know who you are.

- *Do not* smell like smoke or perfume. The client doesn't want your odor lingering in the clothes after the job.

- Please wear deodorant. A smelly model is a bad model.

- No tan lines, no sunburn! Tan lines are not chic, and a lobster face is not ready to work. There is this thing called sunscreen. *Use it.*

- No friends, boyfriends, relatives. This is a job, and you don't go and hang out at their work, so keep them out.

- Guys, wear underwear. No going commando on this one! And do I have to say *wear deodorant* again? Because I mean it!

They don't sugarcoat it for us, because models need to know when they have nasty garlic breath or food in their teeth. We've got makeup people and photographers right in our faces, so bad breath is just rude. It's also not sexy or pretty. And when we just plain stink or show up oblivious to protocol, that's unprofessional. Hearing about our mistakes in such a straightforward way can really make us self-aware, although when we take nitpicking and criticism too personally, self-awareness can lapse into self-consciousness, and that can eventually damage self-esteem. It's a fine line, and tripping over it means you won't be a good model anymore.

Can you spot a self-conscious person when you see one? Can you detect her lack of confidence? Her hunger for approval from others? Can you sense it in her body language and her posture? Sure you can, just like you can spot a self-confident, self-assured person with the nonverbal messages she's sending to the world. For instance, if you're hyperaware of your breath or hair or hemline, you're going to be much less self-aware in terms of your whole self. You'll be hyperfocused, and then you might not notice that you're slumping or that you have a stain on your shirt or that you forgot to brush your teeth or that you've been mainlining junk food all day. You lose your balance. You lose track of Supermodel YOU.

Models are no different. If you walk into a model casting, you can instantly spot the girls who are confident and self-assured just as easily as you can spot the girl who is self-conscious. The confident, self-assured girl will walk into the room with her head held high, shoulders back, core in. She won't just slip into a room. She will arrive. Her pace will be quick, and she will have purpose. A self-conscious model, on the other hand, will walk in a little bit slumped, head down, eyes glancing all over, like she's not even sure why she's there. She'll enter the room tentatively, slowly. She'll sit with hesitation, and she won't meet people's eyes. The confident, self-assured model will do the opposite. She's there for a reason. She's eager, and she's usually more impatient, tapping her foot, legs crossed and swinging (burning calories!), ready to go!

Which one do you want to emulate?

Walking that line between extreme self-consciousness and serene self-awareness can be a challenge. I can't even tell you all the horror stories about being scrutinized as a model. I've had Spanish clients discuss my unattractiveness right in front of me, unaware that I speak fluent Spanish and understood every word. It didn't feel good, of course. But that was their opinion—and every person is entitled to have one—and they obviously didn't think I understood them. Then there was the stylist who refused to do a job if I was the model. He had never even met me, but he hated the way I looked and literally threw the biggest diva fit until they decided to use another girl.

The industry tells me that my face is not commercially beautiful. I have huge, wide-set alien eyes and crooked teeth, and a bunch of other imperfections. Thank God for the success of that movie *Avatar*—I think that's why I keep getting booked! I look just like one of those aliens. When I first started modeling, the *Avatar* look was just about to hit the fashion world. They were still in the baby-doll, little-girl trend, which was never me (not even when I *was* a little girl!). The first time I cast for Armani (the man himself!), he loved me, but he told my agent I had weird eyes! (But then a year later, he had me open his celebrity-packed Armani Privé show!) I was also discovered in Los Angeles, but my agent immediately sent me to New York, and New York sent me to Europe. This was because L.A. is known for commercial work, and your typical, beautiful girl-next-door (this wasn't me, either), and although New York is less commercial than L.A., the look that was "in" at that time wasn't the look I have. Now, with the popularity of *Avatar* and the alien-looking girls, I've had a lot more modeling success.

But what if I had let that criticism stop me at the beginning? Instead, I let it help me become more self-aware. I know how I look, and I know how that's useful in my career—and also how it isn't. It's not always fun, but overall, the criticism I get has helped me more than it's hurt me. I'm glad that my look is unique, like a rare gemstone! That's how I see it. Even if it means some people literally hate the way I look, I'm okay with that. I have to be. Being self-aware means understanding exactly how you look and how people see you, but also seeing the very best in yourself and choosing to embrace it. People can easily take on a self-perception based on how others see them, but I'd rather convince others to see me the way I see myself.

Insecurities and criticism are a part of everyone's life. Nobody is immune. If you use this kind of external judgment to boost your own self-awareness rather than let it tear you down, it can benefit your life in ways you've never imagined. Eventually, you learn who you are, and how that is the same and how it is *not* the same as how other people see you. There is the person you are, and the person you project that you are, and the person you want to be—your higher self or, for the purposes of this book, your supermodel self! The goal of self-awareness is to understand and know the differences among these three selves, and work to unite them. In a perfect world, all of these versions of you would be exactly the same. It's a journey to work toward that, but it's a fun trip to be on—the trip of your life! You will always want more, and you will always be working on maximizing and perfecting your higher self. You are a work in progress, and it's a beautiful journey.

And when you temper your self-awareness with self-compassion, that's when you can develop true self-love and positive self-esteem. Accepting yourself right now, even with all your imperfections, is so important for true self-awareness and fulfillment of all Five Keys. Self-acceptance does not mean settling for your excuses or diminishing your power. It doesn't mean settling for less than you know you deserve. *Au contraire!* With self-awareness, you will be able to identify where you are, and then you get to decide where you want to go. But first, you have to accept and love yourself for who and where you are right now.

SUPERMODEL **SAYS . . .**

I like my butt. It's perfectly proportional, it's cute, and it's still where it belongs. It's been behaving so far, and if it doesn't, I can spank it a little bit and put it back in place, just like I do with my men.

— Joanna Krupa, model/actress appearing on
Dancing with the Stars and *The Real Housewives of Miami*
(as quoted on **www.foxnews.com**)

The example I always use is a modified version of one I heard from Esther and Jerry Hicks, inspirational speakers and authors. Let's say you are on the way to visit me in California! You're driving, and you stop for gas in, say, Arizona. You look around and you see Arizona, and then you get upset that you're still not in California (a metaphor for not yet achieving your goal, like your ideal weight). What are you going to do? Do you just stay in Arizona and say f--- California, because you're obviously not good enough to appear instantaneously in California? Do you turn around and go back to the place you were before, the place you wanted to leave (your unrealized self), because you didn't get to California fast enough? Or do you get back into your car with a full tank of gas and keep going, because you know yourself and you know you can do it? Because you know it takes time to get where you want to go, and that it's a long drive with lots of stops along the way, but you're determined and you have a map and you know your destination? Self-acceptance is trusting yourself and believing that even if you get lost, you will get back on the right road.

It's okay to accept that you aren't at your Supermodel YOU best self yet, but it's also important to know that you *will be*. It doesn't matter that you are currently in Arizona, or that you weigh X number of pounds or that you still don't have your dream job. It doesn't do any good to get mad at Arizona, and it certainly doesn't do any good to get mad at yourself. Acceptance is not *settling.* You aren't going to stay in Arizona. Acceptance is knowing that you are already good enough to keep moving, no matter where your journey has gotten you to this point. Accept who you are, know yourself, love yourself, and then you'll be able to move forward without any barriers, to achieve anything you want—even if what you really want is to head to the *beach,* baby, with a bangin' supermodel bikini body!

MODEL **TALK**

[As a human being] you have all the knowledge within, but you have to make [an] effort to come in touch with that knowledge.

— Swami Rama of the Himalayas

The Self-Awareness Diet

Self-awareness has all kinds of implications for your life, and one of the biggest for the purposes of this book is the way it affects your body, your health, your shape, and your weight. Self-awareness as a weight-loss key is about identifying with your body. This is so important if you really want to achieve the one of your dreams! When you are tuned in to the rhythms, feelings, and changes in your body, you will be better able to identify why you aren't where you want to be. Where is the disconnect between how you want to look and feel, and how you actually look and feel? Where is the self-awareness gap?

That gap is where the action steps go: the things you need to do to get from where you are now to where you want to be. I've read that 95 percent of diets backfire because even if the person loses weight, he or she gains it back, plus a few more pounds. I believe the diet isn't the problem. Most diets work if you follow them. The problem is that you are so stressed-out, with your body constantly in fight-or-flight mode, that anything you eat goes immediately into fat storage. This is a survival mechanism, but it's no way to become Supermodel YOU.

Also, remember what I told you about the law of homeostasis in Chapter 3? Your body fights to regain weight that you lose, and it can take a while to reset your body to your new weight. Self-awareness can help you.

For example, one night recently I went to a Korean spa. I love the Korean spa. They have all these different rooms made of salt, clay, and jade, and they're *hot!* You sweat a lot. There's an ice room, too, but I like to be hot! Anyway, I got home superlate, like around midnight, and I was so relaxed and ready for sleep, but I was starving!

So what did I do? I checked in with the keys: *What the heck, Sarah DeAnna? It's midnight—why do you think you're hungry? You're just tired! Brush your teeth and go to bed!* That's what I thought at first. But I'd probably dropped a pound at the spa, and my body was in major protest mode, so I ended up eating a light snack, then going straight to bed.

Now, this is me. But if you are trying to lose weight, you might have decided: *Hey, I'm tired; I don't need a snack. I could just go to sleep and I'd forget all about this crazy idea that I needed more food today, because I'm self-aware and I know I've had plenty of nutrition. Now what I need is sleep.* Then you could sleep like a baby and wake up feeling light as a feather.

SUPERMODEL **SAYS . . .**

I am always thinner when I am happy and following my dreams, when I don't have time to sit on the couch and worry and eat sweets and feel depressed. When I do feel down, I figure out why, and what I can do to change it. What do I really want to do? Then I make a plan and do it.

— Zdenka Sutton, super–massage therapist, Reiki practitioner, and international model

I have a friend named Roberta. She's a supersweet and beautiful girl who goes to my gym and attends the same classes I do, and more. I swear that every time I go to the gym or any yoga studio, she's always there! These are hard-core cardio and body-sculpting classes. You burn a bazillion calories, and they *will* leave you with a pretty nice bod . . . unless you are like Roberta (and a lot of other people at the gym and in my classes). She is probably 30 pounds overweight, hates her body, is totally stressed-out all the time, and has a poor self-image. It's heartbreaking to me and confusing to her.

We've all seen a Roberta (or a "Robert") who has the same story. Roberta practically lives at the gym, has a personal trainer, and can probably out-stamina me on any given day. But she's not channeling her inner supermodel.

So what exactly is going on here? We already know from the first chapter that we can't blame genetics, although Roberta definitely uses that as an excuse. However, I don't believe that's her problem. After talking to Roberta, I discovered a number of reasons why she's not at her Supermodel YOU ideal physique. She's not practicing the Five Keys:

- Roberta only *sleeps* four or five hours a night. She claims that's all she needs.

- Roberta usually skips breakfast and doesn't *eat* until lunch. (She says she eats really healthy food. I believe her and don't think her diet is the problem.)

- Roberta has a high-*stress* job.

- Roberta says she needs to *work out* to avoid getting fat. She takes yoga to calm and center herself, since she's always stressed-out.

First and foremost, she isn't following the *first* key, and without the first key, it's almost impossible to follow all the others. If Roberta were truly self-aware, she would know she needed more sleep than four or five hours, because she would feel it in her body. She is not tuned in to how her body is really doing with her routine.

If Roberta slept more, her stress hormones wouldn't be running wild the way they obviously are. Even with the yoga she does, she's still overdoing it. She's asking an awful lot out of her little yoga class. Yoga alone can only go so far in defusing your stress response, and some kinds of yoga and other exercise actually create more stress, especially if you do too much. Roberta should balance all those workouts with some meditation, in addition to more sleep.

If Roberta gave her body food in the morning when it requires it, her body would understand that she wasn't starving, and it would stop storing every single thing she ate as fat. Breakfast is so crucial! Your body will tell you this if you can get past defaulting to your bad habit of skipping the first meal of the day. I know breakfast isn't for everyone—some people really don't like to eat it, and in some cases I think that can be okay—but if you work out in the morning, you have to give your body some fuel or you will seriously deplete yourself! Also, if you don't eat food when your body needs energy, you're likely to overeat later in the day, and that can add up to way more calories than a simple, healthy breakfast would have added. Studies have also shown that students who eat breakfast perform better on morning tests. Breakfast fuels your body *and* your brain.

I actually never used to eat breakfast, but then I met this beautiful, thin, healthy woman who swore by it. I told her how I wasn't hungry in the morning, and she explained to me that she isn't either, but that breakfast, like most things in life, is a habit. I decided to try it, and now it's a habit for me, too. And I feel better throughout the day.

Finally, Roberta does enough exercise to power a small factory, but she's overworking her body, which is causing more stress, which is probably making her sleep even less. The bottom line is that this lack of self-awareness is resulting in a thunder butt instead of a yoga butt.

With just a little Supermodel YOU insight, Roberta could become more self-aware, improve her sleep habits, be able to eat more and exercise less . . . and she would be so much less stressed! She would have more time and energy to spend on just being happy with herself and her body, instead of feeling chained to the gym. And then I would bet money her excess weight would start to come off. With just a few "key" changes, Roberta could relax right into her dream body, find the life of her dreams, and live happily ever after. If she ever asks for my help, that's exactly what I will tell her. (I let people come to me when they are ready.)

Self-Awareness Leads to Self-Control

Like most people, I have a couple of food addictions—things I love and tend to overeat if I'm not being self-aware. Mine are mainly for healthy things like carrots (I know, sometimes I think I'm so strange!), but when I overeat carrots, even though they probably won't make me fat, they do make my skin turn orange. The fact is that *anything* is unhealthy if it becomes an addiction, whether it's French fries or spinach. Even exercise can become an addiction. Of course, it's better to be addicted to carrots than, say, heroin . . . but self-awareness is a far better option than both, and self-awareness is exactly what can help you conquer your personal food (and other) demons.

I recently spoke at a conference, and one of the other speakers was self-help guru Wayne Dyer. During the event, he was talking about his daughter getting sober from drugs, and he said, "We are all addicts. She does yoga three times a day now." She had replaced her unhealthy addiction with a healthier one, but it was still an addiction. A healthier addiction can be a good way to step down from an unhealthy one, but as you are moving in the right direction, self-awareness is where you're headed.

This brings me to the issue of self-control. One of the reasons I hear cited most often by people who can't seem to do what they know they should do to get healthy and lose extra weight is that they have no self-control. But self-control is just part of self-awareness. When you aren't self-aware, self-control seems impossible. When you are self-aware, self-control becomes much more attainable. When you're totally tuned in to how your bad habits affect your body and mind, then you will logically want to stop the bad effects, and you will directly experience how bad effects result from bad choices, and how good effects result from good choices. And then you can decide, with a rational mind, what to do—rather than with an addiction-addled mind that feels swept away by outside forces and isn't self-aware.

For example, if you mindlessly power through a pint of ice cream, then you're probably going to mindlessly *not* notice how bloated and low on energy and heavy you feel. But if you are self-aware, then even if you eat the ice cream, you might be questioning yourself about why. *Why did I do that? What did I get out of it that I needed? What did I get out of it that I <u>didn't</u> need or want? Was it worth it? Let me weigh the pros and cons.* If the bad effects, short-term and long-term, aren't worth the ice cream, then next time, although you might not pass on the ice cream, you might give it a second thought, and decide to notice some more about what it does to you. And the time after that, maybe you'll just have a couple of spoonfuls, really taste it, really savor it, and then stop. Or you might even pass. Or decide ice cream doesn't really fit so well into your new Supermodel YOU lifestyle.

The beautiful thing about the first key is that *I'm not telling you not to eat ice cream.* But I am telling you to recognize whether or not *you* really want to eat the ice cream, and whether you really will *decide* to eat the ice cream or decide not to eat it.

Cravings mean something, and it isn't always what you think, if you aren't practicing self-awareness. Doreen Virtue, superauthor and angel therapist, wrote about this in her great book *Constant Craving.* She talks about the real underlying cravings behind food cravings, and I see her theories playing out all the time in the people I know. For example, one of my best friends isn't 100 percent happy with her weight, and whenever I ask her why she thinks her weight is so difficult for her, she says that she just loves fried, fatty foods and can't help it! That's her main excuse for not being at her ideal weight. Her rationale is that she loves fatty food, and fatty food makes her happy, and since I'm such a fan of happy, who am I to tell her to give up something she loves?

My friend is self-aware enough to know her problem area. Most people are. They know they're suckers for chocolate or pizza or cheese or whatever it is. If they think they're just lazy and that's why they never get any exercise, they'll often readily admit it, but they stop there and accept that. They don't *investigate* the impulse for chocolate or laziness with self-awareness. What the first key asks you to do, however, is to go deep into those places where you think you are weak or you think you fail. Apply self-awareness to those places. Sit quietly and just think about it, without letting yourself get distracted by other things. Give it some focused time and see what comes up.

Doreen Virtue says that when people crave fat, they are actually hiding from fear. "Often, the high-fat eater is deeply afraid of something. Of being alone. Of facing a terrible truth. Of taking responsibility. Of making changes. These fears and insecurities are quelled by a consistently plugged stomach." If this is true, and I believe it is, then a dose of self-awareness might help my friend to get to the bottom of her cravings for fatty foods. Instead of just saying, "I love fatty foods—the end," she could say, "*Why* do I love fatty foods? Does this say something about me? Am I missing something in my life? Do I need to face something?"

This applies to every area of your life that isn't going the way you want it to. Don't just accept it or complain about it. Get to the bottom of it! Use self-awareness, and consider yourself your own greatest experiment. Ask *why.* Do you need more love? More affection? More energy? More job satisfaction? Is your self-esteem suffering?

You won't always know the answer to the question *Why?* At least, not at first. But self-awareness will help you find it eventually, and it's going to be well worth the search.

Of course, models have an advantage when it comes to body self-awareness, because our jobs depend on keeping our physiques looking good. Think about what you prioritize. Do you refuse to let anything get in the way of your career, but then you neglect your body? Are you a fierce Mama Bear with your kids, but refuse to defend yourself against criticism and negative self-esteem?

To make self-awareness work, you have to *put yourself first*. This is the whole point. It's the only way you'll ever be any good to anyone else, so it's not really selfish at all. If your health and the achievement of your dreams come first, you won't have to resent anybody, you won't overeat when you don't really want that extra food, and you'll achieve balance, which includes losing excess weight you've been lugging around. It's an awesome and exciting process, and you can start *right now!* Just act like a supermodel. *You can't be overweight. You can't have less than the best body possible. It's your job. Your life depends on it.* Believe it. No more excuses for barreling through your life on autopilot without noticing you've got a stain on your shirt, spinach between your teeth, or a cupcake in one hand and a cheeseburger in the other. Enough! Excuses diminish your power and your purpose. You are in charge now. You're Supermodel YOU!

A self-aware person can understand why things happen to her. She knows when she's really hungry, and when she's eating out of boredom or anxiety or because she didn't get enough sleep. You might still eat out of boredom. You might not always get enough sleep. But if you are self-aware, you will *realize this,* and not use it as an excuse to make it worse. You won't blame someone else. And you won't keep spiraling downward. You'll be able to stop yourself before you go too far because you actually noticed which way you were going. It's incredibly empowering to know that you are in control of *you.*

MODEL **TALK**

Fifty percent of the brain is dedicated to vision. How you look plays a large role in how you feel. Both matter to your success at work and in your relationships. It is not just vanity, it is about health. To look and feel your best, you must first think about and optimize your brain.

— Daniel G. Amen, M.D., superpsychiatrist and
New York Times best-selling author
(from *Change Your Brain, Change Your Body*)

The Upside of Vanity

Maybe you think that too much attention to your appearance is vain, but vanity has an upside. Without vanity, we might not shower, wear deodorant, brush our hair or teeth, or get that joy that comes from getting dressed up and looking pretty. A lot of models are vain, but in many ways, that sets the stage for the rest of the Five Keys to fall into place. Vanity can plant the seed of commitment toward your body. Your body is the vehicle for your spirit. That's worth taking care of! That's worth noticing.

Self-awareness helps you be more tuned in to how you look. When was the last time you looked in the mirror? If you look in the mirror every five minutes, then you probably need to spend more time focusing on how you feel *inside*—maybe you've crossed the line into self-consciousness. But if you haven't actually "seen" yourself lately, maybe it's time to check in.

Your outside is a reflection of your inside. Not in every way— I'm not judging your body type, your hairstyle, your clothing choices. But if you are sloppy, careless, unkempt, slouching, slinking around like you're ashamed of yourself, sitting hunched over, scowling, or otherwise looking completely unplugged from your physical body, then you need a self-awareness wake-up call. And if you are strong, confident, beautiful, and powerful at any weight and in any clothing, you will look like a supermodel! You will be gorgeous.

Appearance will make a difference in the way the world treats you, too, whether that's right or wrong. Pretty children are generally more popular with both friends and teachers in school, and tend to get better grades and more positive attention. Pretty people are more likely to get jobs and get paid more for those jobs, are found guilty in court less often (and when they are found guilty, they receive lighter sentences), and are just generally treated better in life. This may sound totally unfair to you, and it is! Appearance isn't everything. On the other hand, people who take pride in how they look and make the most of it can reap all these benefits. It's not necessarily natural traits that give you the advantage or the disadvantage. It's what you do with what you've got. That's just one more incentive to look your supermodel best!

Modeltude

If part of self-awareness is loving the body you're finally paying more attention to, another part is to adjust your attitude when your self-awareness reveals that your attitude sucks. This is one of the most important things about cultivating self-awareness: it gives you the opportunity to change how you see things. For example, a lot of models truly believe they can eat anything they want and not get fat. They say (and think!) things like, "I can eat anything I want. I'm just naturally thin." And it becomes true! You are your thoughts. You know that old quote "I think, therefore I am"? The Supermodel YOU version is: "What I think, I am."

MODEL **TALK**

People should think about what they think about. You become what you think.

— Ryan Blair, supersuccessful serial entrepreneur,
New York Times best-selling author, and business "supermodel"

Another thing models do that a lot of successful people do (I read that most successful CEOs and leaders do this) is dissociate from failures. So, say I go to a casting and don't book the job. The modeling world has taught me that it has nothing to do with me. Maybe they wanted a brunette. Or maybe they wanted a girl who had fuller hair or dark eyes or whatever. Or maybe the other model and I didn't look good together. Or maybe they wanted an Asian or Latina look. A healthy modeltude is to not get down on yourself because you didn't book the job, or didn't do whatever you were trying to do. Modeltude means feeling great about yourself, no matter the external circumstances. When failure happens (which it will eventually, to everyone), to have modeltude is to depersonalize the experience.

So, say you get rejected by a guy or don't get the job you wanted—you know, the things that freak you out and make you doubt yourself and possibly overeat? Depersonalize it. Depersonalize anything negative (but personalize everything positive, like when you hear complimentary words such as *beauty, hot, gorgeous, strong,* and *pretty*). Because the bad stuff probably isn't about you anyway. Maybe the guy isn't over his last relationship. Maybe the job required someone with a particular skill set that isn't exactly yours. That's not your fault. That guy and that job wouldn't have been right for you anyway, so thank goodness it didn't work out! You're better than to settle for a situation that's not right for you. The so-called rejection has *nothing* to do with how incredible you are as a person, inside and out.

Depersonalizing isn't the same as lacking self-awareness. The self-aware person will recognize if the rejection is related to something she did, and then she can consider how she might alter her behavior or whatever it is, if that works for her. But she doesn't get all hurt or upset by it, because she knows that it has nothing to do with her higher self. Any other attitude will just stress you out (see Key 3!).

Another thing models do: pretend other people are thinking great things about you, instead of believing they are thinking anything negative. Why not? You don't really know what other people are thinking anyway, so why assume the worst? Why not assume the best? Models really are often being judged and picked apart, and that can wear on us after a while, so it's a good self-esteem booster to think things like, *She may be criticizing my walk, but deep down, she's thinking how much she admires my legs!* In general, in the modeling world and outside of it, people are a lot more concerned with themselves than they are with you. It's true! So whenever you think people are judging you or talking about you, or even if they look at you funny, just decide that they're thinking good things, and send them good thoughts back. Karma, baby!

MODEL **TALK**

Be careful what you pretend to be because you are what you pretend to be.

— Kurt Vonnegut, super–sci-fi writer and awesome visionary

When I first started modeling and was in Paris, my agency treated me like a supermodel. (This was a different agency from the one that put me up in that horrible New York apartment I told you about before.) They took me to fancy dinners and lavish parties, arranged for drivers to pick me up and take me home, spoke highly of me to others, introduced me to important people in my industry, put me up in the nicer of their two model apartments (a beautiful flat in Saint-Germain near the Seine), and so on. Their theory was "If we want to make you a supermodel, then we're going to treat you like a supermodel." I never forgot that.

You might not have anybody wining and dining you at the moment, but you can totally do this for yourself. If you want to have the body of your dreams, act as if you already do, and treat yourself as if you do. Cherish and treasure your perfect body! It's not about vanity; it's about self-love and self-respect.

I really got to see this in action the first time I ever went to a show casting. This was a major *Aha* moment for me when it comes to the way a person's outer self reflects the inner self, because I was able to witness several models walk (that is, audition for the runway job) and get picked apart in front of me. I was fascinated by what the designer said about the models—every little thing, from how they held their arms and where they placed their feet to how their hair looked, how the clothes fit them, and how they looked when they moved. Of course it made me so ridiculously self-conscious that by the time it was my turn to walk for the designer, I was so filled with nerves and anxiety that I totally blew it. But at least I was acutely aware of everything I was doing. In fact, this was my state of mind for my first full fashion circuit: fashion shows in New York, Milan, and Paris. I went to more than

100 castings and had to walk 100 or more times for designers, and every time, I was such a nervous wreck! My legs were shaking, my heart was racing, my face was beet red . . . no wonder I didn't book any shows!

But it was a great lesson for me. At that first casting, the designer was really rude, and she made girls walk several times and scrutinized everything about them. There was one beautiful model who walked with such confidence and was so debonair (she was a veteran model). I thought she was great and was sure to book the job. To my surprise, the designer kept having her walk and pointing out every imperfection. For example, she swung her right arm, but not her left arm. I never even noticed that. Ever since then, I became crazy-conscientious of my every step, my posture, my stride, how my arms swing, and so on. Had I not been a model, I probably never would have consciously questioned these things, but it did something to my self-awareness. It heightened it, and it made me a better model, even if some of those initial criticisms stung a little bit.

This is what I mean by supermodel body awareness! It might not be your job to know these things, but aren't you at all curious to know if you turn your right foot out more than your left when you walk or if your shoulders cave inward, telling not only everyone you meet but also own body that you lack confidence? Tweaking these external parts of yourself can make huge differences in what's going on inside.

MODEL **TALK**

If you change your physiology—that is, your posture, breathing patterns, muscle tension, facial expressions, gestures, movements, words, vocal tonality—you instantly change your internal representations and your state.

— Anthony Robbins, superinspirational self-help guru

And then there is the other side of it: how you treat others. That designer might have just been doing her job, trying to get the absolute most out of the models. Or maybe she was an unhappy person, taking out her negativity on them. That's her problem, not yours, not mine. Everyone is responsible for their own state of mind. And I always look for the beauty in everyone I see. Always! When I meet people, I almost always compliment them on what it was that I noticed, from their hair to their perfect smile or whatever it is that caught my eye. When you approach life like that, that's what life will give you back. It makes people happy, and then they really *are* more likely to say and think good things about you. It's a win-win. When you look for the beauty in others, the beauty in yourself will reflect back.

If you learn to change your attitude, you can change your life, not just your pants size. Models know that their thoughts are very powerful. Instead of wasting time like most people do beating themselves up and sabotaging their own bodies and minds, models use their thoughts to feel good about themselves.

Here are some examples of how you might think about things now, and how you can modelize your thoughts:

> **You:** Ugh. Not only do I look terrible, but I look fat, too! I am so fat.
> **A model:** I'm, like, so friggin' hot! And I have a smokin' body!

> **You:** Great. Just great. That chocolate cake is going straight to my butt!
> **A model:** I eat whatever I want, and I never gain a pound. [Eating just a few delicious bites.]

> **You:** I hate exercising, and I totally don't have the time. I'll never be skinny, because I hate to go to the gym!
> **A model:** I don't need to exercise. I'm on the move all the time.

You: I'm just naturally a bigger girl. It's genetic.
A model: What can I say? I'm just naturally gorgeous!

You: I feel so fat and ugly.
A model: I feel so sexy. Everybody notices how great
I look.

You: I wish I were prettier.
A model: I am beautiful. Everybody sees it.

SUPERMODEL **SAYS . . .**

*I eat throughout the day, as much as I want, when I want,
whatever I want. Honestly, I just listen to my body and eat what
I'm craving that day.*

— Taylor Reynolds, superauthentic model,
represented by Muse Model Management, New York

Here are a few more tricks I use for cultivating modeltude.
Please steal them!

— **Use images.** Whenever I see pictures in magazines or online that make me feel good or powerful, I cut them out or print
them out and hang them around my house. Then, whenever I see
these images, I feel good, powerful, and strong, and I get into a
positive frame of mind.

— **Personalize positive words.** Every time I hear someone say
words like *beautiful, pretty,* or *great body,* I pretend the person is
talking about me. I just tell myself, *There they go, talking about me
again!* It might sound silly, but it's fun, and it's a great mood booster, especially when you realize they're really talking about a sports
car or a painting. You can do this with all positive words you hear
out there in the world: *gorgeous* (a sunset?), *flawless* (a diamond?),
nice rack (a bike rack?), *hot* (cup of coffee at Starbucks?). It doesn't

matter what *they* are talking about. Just personalize it. Internalize it. Let it be about you. I even do this in yoga class, like when the teacher is saying "Beautiful pose" to someone else, I pretend he said it to me. Do this whenever you hear someone else being praised at school, at work, at home, wherever. It will make you feel like all is well—and then it all *will* be well.

— **Pretend.** Start acting like you already have a supermodel body. You are *already* Supermodel YOU! Do it by talking, walking, and acting like a model (this book is full of examples for you to emulate, when the spirit moves you). Whether you are walking into your office or dropping your kids off at school, do it with confidence and beauty. Part of getting there is acting like you are *already* there! You're faking it 'til you make it. All models do this, so why shouldn't you? Frequently remind yourself that supermodels aren't born, they're made.

— **Develop model posture.** Just changing your posture, your facial expression, and the way you walk or sit can totally change how you feel inside. It's transformation from the outside in! Try it. When you are feeling blah or insecure, stand up straight, roll your shoulders back, hold your head up high, tighten your core, and walk with swagger. Keep it up and you'll start to feel more confident and beautiful. It's like magic! As a recent Cole Haan campaign states, "Strut, don't stroll!" So strut it, baby!

— **Cultivate a modeltourage.** When models hang out together in a big group, we call it a modeltourage. You can have one, too. Studies show that you tend to take on the habits, and also the weight issues, of the people you hang around with, so find a group of friends who inspire you, motivate you, and provide positive support for your Supermodel YOU journey. Hang out with them often. Your own personal modeltourage!

— **Assume the best.** Whenever I get a little insecure or start to think that people are talking about me in a bad way (like at castings), I pretend that they are whispering to each other about how incredible and amazing I am. I watch their faces, even if I can't hear what they're saying, and I imagine the whole conversation going something like this: "That Sarah DeAnna is incredible. I've never seen a model with such complex and unique beauty. We've got to do whatever we can to get her onto this campaign. Offer her more money! We'll pay any price!" Maybe it sounds vain (I am a model, after all), but it sure beats the alternative, like assuming they are whispering about how badly my dress fits or how they can't believe I'm not wearing any makeup or how much they hate my shoes. Assuming the opposite totally works! I dare you to try it!

MODEL **TALK**

I don't at all like knowing what people say of me behind my back. It makes me far too conceited.

— Oscar Wilde, superplaywright (from *An Ideal Husband*)

Self-Awareness Matters

If I haven't convinced you by now that self-awareness is the avenue to changing anything and everything about yourself, I'm going to have to pull out the Santa Claus metaphor. Sorry, but you made me do it!

Do you remember when you found out Santa Claus wasn't real? You were probably a little devastated and upset at first. *I* was. But eventually, you laugh at yourself for really believing in Santa, his team of flying reindeer, and all those little elves up in the North Pole. You know that it's not even possible to fly from California to Australia overnight, so how in the world could Mr. Claus possibly cart a sleigh around the globe on Christmas Eve? Slide down millions of chimneys? And leave *all* those presents for *all* those kids?

Somehow, all along, you *knew,* even though you didn't actually *know.*

But once you became aware that Santa doesn't, in fact, exist (at least not literally . . . I'm not trying to spoil anybody's Christmas spirit, or offend anyone of a different religion—it's just an analogy—and OMG, if you still believe in Santa, I am *supersorry!*), everything changed. You were able to figure out how all those presents got under your tree. Why, it was your parents all along!

Your weight or any other thing you don't like about your appearance is just the same. You were told or just decided that all these things about your body were true. You had a story about yourself and your body: what you should weigh, how much you eat versus how much you *should* eat, how much you are supposed to exercise, how big your thighs are destined to be . . . all of that. But what if everything you thought was true was just a made-up story, like the myth that Santa Claus comes down your chimney with a sackful of presents on Christmas Eve?

The only way to really make a difference in your weight, not to mention in your personal happiness, is to *know.* You have to become self-aware or you'll never know the truth about why you gained extra weight or why you're tired all the time, or why you just don't feel like you're living as well and as happily as you could be. You won't understand why you don't have the body of your dreams and why you can't seem to get it. Self-awareness is where it all begins.

People are aware that eating too much fast food will probably make them fat, that smoking cigarettes causes lung cancer and heart attacks, and that stressing out is bad for their health. But a lot of people still do these things. Why?

Self-awareness is the key to knowing why, and then knowing what would fix the problem for *you* if you aren't living the way you want to live, feeling the way you want to feel, or looking the way you really want to look. Self-awareness is the key to the self-esteem and the self-love that will urge you to do what feels good for you, and what is nourishing and compassionate for your body. You need to value *you,* and you can't do that until you know what you're worth to yourself. And that takes self-awareness.

SUPERMODEL **PLAYLIST**

Country music just makes me feel like me. That's how music <u>should</u> make you feel. Like you find little pieces of yourself in each song. These are some of my favorite country songs:

Luke Bryan, "Drunk on You"
Jason Aldean, "Dirt Road Anthem"
Little Big Town, "Pontoon"
Rascal Flatts, "No Reins"
Craig Campbell, "Fish"
Hunter Hayes, "Wanted"
Jerrod Niemann, "Lover, Lover"
Josh Turner, "Would You Go with Me"
Jason Aldean, "She's Country"
Kenny Chesney, "Somewhere with You"

— Lacey James, veteran working model

So let's cultivate some self-awareness and talk about *you*. Let's play "20 Questions." No matter how self-aware you are right now, you can always cultivate more. Answer these questions for yourself. Take as much time as you need. Discuss them with your friends. Write them down. Talk them over. Use them to become more self-aware.

- How tall are you?

- How much do you weigh? (Be honest with yourself. You don't have to tell anyone else.)

- How much would you *like* to weigh? Do you think that's a realistic goal for you?

- What is your dream body, aside from what anyone has told you it should be? What is it to *you?*

- What are your strengths? Your best features? Your best personality traits?

- What are your weaknesses? The things you don't like about yourself? The things you would like to change?

- How do your friends describe you? Do you agree with their descriptions? Why or why not?

- What are some of the things you believe about your body and your ability to improve it?

- When you think about your inner dialogue, or the way you talk to yourself, what tone do you usually use? Do you tend to be self-critical, or do you try to boost your own mood or motivation?

- List two situations when you have been most at ease. What specific elements were present when you felt that way?

- What types of activities did you enjoy doing when you were a child? What about now?

- What motivates you? Why?

- What are your dreams for the future? What steps are you taking to achieve your dreams?

- What do you fear most in your life? Why?

- Where do you think you could use some improvement in your habits?

- What are you really getting right at this time in your life?

- What stresses you? What is your typical response to stress?

- What qualities do you like to see in people? Why?

- Do most of your friends have the qualities you like to see in people? Why or why not?

- When you disagree with someone's viewpoint, what do you do?

We'll go more into this kind of self-examination in Chapter 9, but for now, these questions are really just practice for honing your inner voice, so that it helps build you up instead of tearing you down. Your inner voice should be positive and reassuring. For people with low self-esteem, the inner voice becomes a harsh inner critic, constantly deriding, punishing, and belittling their accomplishments. The better you know and understand yourself, the more compassion you will have for yourself, and that's when your inner voice can become your cheerleader rather than your critic. This is all part of using self-awareness to your own benefit.

How Self-Awareness Leads to Self-Actualization

Finally, I want to talk about how self-awareness can take you way beyond a supermodel body and into superconsciousness, or self-actualization. Self-actualization, the way I use it, is the full realization of your potential. This is basic psychology stuff—that self-actualization is the primary human drive. But I think it's something more—it's also complete self-acceptance and self-love. It's that state where you realize there is nothing wrong with you, even as you continually strive to perfect yourself.

Self-actualization goes beyond body, even beyond mind. It's the place where you know yourself completely, and in that complete knowing, you are able to achieve your own perfection. You become the best version of yourself, not just in your own mind, but in reality. You become actualized—fully and completely you, which is to say perfect. The famous psychologist Abraham Maslow defined *self-actualization* as the full realization of one's potential based on what is already inside you. It doesn't come from the outside, and it is based in growth rather than deficiency. I like that. I think that's completely true.

I often say that when it comes to body image, most of us have an ideal version of ourselves in our heads, which basically means we hold a picture of our desired physical selves that we would like to achieve. Yet, we spend so much time punishing ourselves for not having achieved it yet. We spend so much time and energy on feeling unhappy and stressed about our physical bodies. But the mistake is in thinking we are deficient. No, that body image we have exists as a reality within each one of us, and when we become self-actualized—when we love and embrace who we are—that's when we truly free up our time, energy, and resources so that we can actually fulfill our potential. That's when we can make it happen. We don't have to go out and get it. All we have to do is realize it and then manifest it.

MODEL **TALK**

Knowing others is wisdom, knowing yourself is enlightenment.

— Lao-tzu, superphilosopher and founder of Taoism

Life is a process of working toward self-actualization. It doesn't matter if you aren't there yet. Hardly anybody is. Who can say they have already achieved their full potential? This is the work of a lifetime, but it's a goal we can all work toward, and practicing the Five Keys is a way down the path. Nurture your body, and your mind will be set free to achieve anything. This is where we're headed. But we've got some more work to do first, so let's move on to Key 2!

■ ■ ■

CHAPTER FIVE

Key 2: Beauty Sleep

We've all heard the phrase "sleep your way to the top." But now we've got a new take on that—the right way to do it, that is.

— *CBS News* REPORT ON GETTING ADEQUATE SLEEP

Let's pretend for a minute that you're a model and you have a photo shoot tomorrow morning. Why not? You're on the way to your supermodel body, so play the part, at least in your own mind. Pretend your agency just called you to confirm that you'll be shooting a beauty story that's going to run in *Elle* magazine next month with one of the world's most famous photographers, and your call time is 6 A.M. That means you need to be there at 6 A.M., which means you have to be up by at least 4:30 A.M. to get there on time. Ugh! Models hate early call times, and being late is totally stressful!

Shooting for beauty basically involves just your face, photographed at close range. That means that the camera is going to be zoomed in on every little pore and imperfection. It's roughly 6 P.M. now. It's Friday night, and you've already made plans with the girls to go out dancing, but because models don't typically receive their call sheet for the next day until 5 or 6 P.M., you didn't have any idea that you'd be working. Now you know, and you've got a decision to make. You know what your skin looks like when you don't get enough sleep: the shade, the texture, the circles under your eyes, the puffiness. Do you still go out? Or do you cancel?

Contrary to public perception (as I discussed when I dismissed all those nasty model myths), if you really were a model and this actually was your reality, you'd almost certainly cancel your plans and stay home and make sure you got your beauty sleep, especially if you were shooting beauty. This is a big reason why people think models are flaky, but it's not because we just randomly change our minds about our plans. We have good reason! When doing a runway show, a fashion shoot, or just a fitting, a model will almost always choose beauty sleep over everything else in the name of vanity and looking good.

SUPERMODEL **SAYS . . .**

Sleep is so important! I do my best to get eight hours a night and often take naps in the afternoon when possible.

— Heather Chantal Jones, supersweet, wholesome model
and *America's Next Top Model* runner-up

I'm actually a terrible sleeper! Horrible! I sleep really lightly. Caffeine after noon will keep me up all night. A car door slamming five blocks away will jolt me out of my beauty sleep. When I have a restless night, I always notice that the next day, I am:

- Tired
- Overeating
- Craving sugar
- Less energetic and less likely to modercize (let alone exercise!)
- Moody
- More self-critical, with lower self-esteem

But seeing and knowing all of that is a huge step in the right direction (self-awareness!). The brownie might still win, but I'll probably only have some of it, not three of them. Self-awareness keeps my eating in check, even when I'm not at my best. Of course, even better would be to consistently get enough beauty sleep.

Why Sleep Makes You Pretty

We all need beauty sleep (at least seven and a half hours, according to the National Sleep Foundation; the average woman only gets six). And being well rested is directly related to being Supermodel YOU. Models need beauty sleep to be beautiful! We know that skimping on ZZZs will definitely show up on the face one way or another. When we snooze, our bodies go into repair mode to regenerate our skin. This is why the term *beauty sleep* isn't just a catchy little phrase. It's literally true.

During this regeneration time, new skin cells replace old, dead skin, resulting in a fresher-looking face (the kind not just models but *every* person wants). This happens more quickly at night compared to daytime, says Alex Khadavi, M.D., associate dermatology professor at the University of Southern California. Here's some background: Cell turnover gets into high gear at about 2 A.M. when there is a surge in growth hormone. If you are settled into a nice, deep beauty sleep that began at, say, 11 P.M., your face gets rejuvenated. If you are awake all night, your body won't be in healing mode, so it can't take advantage of this growth-hormone surge to repair daily damage from UV rays and pollution and, especially for models, the layers upon layers of makeup spackled onto our skin.

Without your beauty sleep, you won't look as good. Period. A model can't afford to let that happen. Showing up looking and feeling tired is totally unacceptable when your job and your paycheck depend on you taking a pretty picture. But let's be honest— showing up looking and feeling tired doesn't do *you* any good, either. You may have a big presentation or that key job interview or even a major date the next day. Or you might just want to feel good, be productive, and enjoy your day. You can't do that walking around like a zombie because you stayed up all night watching TV or going out, even though you knew you had to get up early. Looking and feeling tired can ruin any important moment, and in the scheme of things, life is full of important moments. What if you have one tomorrow and you don't even know it's coming? Don't you want to be ready? Don't you want to be alert and looking gorgeous?

Think about it: How many times has someone said to you, "You look tired"? It's an insult, I know, but sometimes you can't deny the truth. Lack of beauty sleep really does show up on your face as more wrinkles, less radiant skin, dark circles under the eyes, uneven complexion, more frown and tension lines—and in a lot of other unattractive ways. A makeup artist can only do so much. We know beauty sleep makes us pretty.

Why Supermodel YOU Needs Beauty Sleep

But here's another reason why you need beauty sleep—not sleeping can make you fat. That's right, I said it: *fat.* It's the second beauty-sleep biggie: if a model runs up a debt in her beauty-sleep bank, she is going to overeat, and that means good-bye to her supermodel body and good looks (and *adios* to work, paychecks, and supermodel stardom).

Studies show that people tend to weigh more if they beauty-sleep less. Researchers at Columbia University found that people who slept six hours per night were 23 percent more likely to be obese than people who slept between seven and nine hours. Need more? A study from Case Western Reserve University found that women who slept five or fewer hours per night were 32 percent more likely to experience major weight gain than those who slept an average of seven hours.

Wait, there's more still! At Harvard University, researchers tracked 68,000 women and found that those who clocked only five or fewer hours of rest a night had a 32 percent greater chance of gaining more than 30 pounds over a 16-year period than those who got seven hours of sleep. And most recently, the University of Chicago Sleep Research Lab reported that study subjects who got a full night's sleep (eight and a half hours) burned more fat than those who slept for five and a half hours. OMG, this beauty-sleep business is for real!

Nerd Alert!

What's the connection between lack of beauty sleep and over-eating? Scientists don't know for sure, but there are many theories. Like less time in bed leads you to be both tired and hungry, thanks to a funny-sounding hormone called *ghrelin*. I always say that not sleeping enough brings out the *ghremlin!* (I personally turn into a monster when I don't get enough sleep!) According to sleep expert Michael Breus, M.D., the bodies of sleep-deprived women are high in ghrelin (the hormone that stimulates hunger and promotes fat retention) and low in leptin (the hormone that says to your body, "You're full and can stop eating"). Plus, not only do you want *more* food when you're sleep-deprived, you also want junkier food; your body craves simple carbohydrates (chocolate, pastries, candy) that it can break down fast for quick energy. When you skip beauty sleep, you feel stressed, pig out, and get caught in a calorie-packed cycle.

Also, when you don't get enough sleep, your body is in a chronic state of stress. That jacks up your cortisol levels (one of the main stress hormones in your body that signals high alert), and also messes with your insulin levels, which tells your body that it had better start storing fat, just in case the emergency results in starvation. This is all bad news for your supermodel body, which won't be a supermodel body for long if you keep depriving it of the beauty sleep it truly needs!

And if you go to bed at 10 or 11, you won't be noshing at midnight. You do the math. Umm . . . *hello!* This is a total no-brainer. Sleep more, weigh less! Duh! This is probably the easiest key to channeling your inner supermodel.

Sleeping well and being Supermodel YOU are both natural, and they depend on one another. If you don't beauty-sleep properly, there is almost no way you can maintain a healthy weight (let alone be a pleasant, functioning person). In fact, if you add one hour of beauty sleep to your sweet skinny dreams, you could drop 14 pounds! A study from the University of Michigan shows that you'll likely eat 6 percent less if you replace 60 minutes of awake time (when you may snack unnecessarily) with an hour of shut-eye.

It makes me crazy that so many people claim to need only a few hours of beauty sleep a night. In fact, people praise and admire them for it! People say, "I can sleep when I'm dead," but not sleeping will make you *feel* dead when you should feel *alive!* Sleep deprivation affects your entire system. I've yet to meet one of these four- or five-hour sleepers who is skealthy. You simply cannot fight nature, and nature says we need beauty sleep!

Some people even call sleep a "luxury." Luxury? Please! To say that we don't need sleep is like saying we don't need water, air, food, or iPhones. Absurd! Beauty sleep is essential to our existence; it is a necessity, not a luxury.

According to Kristen Hairston, M.D., a researcher at Wake Forest University School of Medicine in Winston-Salem, North Carolina, people don't usually understand the many ways in which lack of sleep affects them. In her recent study, Dr. Hairston found that people under 40 who slept five hours or less had 32 percent more belly fat than those who got an average of six or seven hours of beauty sleep. And girls, belly fat does not look good in a bikini! But it's not just how you look that's at stake: that excess pooch is not only going to prevent you from achieving your supermodel body, but it can also increase your risk of diabetes and high blood pressure.

On top of all that, sleep deprivation can cause major problems in your life. According to the National Highway Traffic Safety Administration, fatigue causes 100,000 auto crashes and 1,500 crash-related deaths every year in the U.S., most often for people under 25 years old. Sleep deprivation was also a factor in some of the worst disasters in history, including the nuclear accidents at Three Mile Island and Chernobyl, and the huge *Exxon Valdez* oil spill.

I've also read that sleep deprivation makes you dumber, and no model can afford that! We need all the brainpower we can get, and we can't exactly afford to lose any! We certainly don't need the impaired attention, concentration, reasoning, problem solving, and alertness that come with not getting enough beauty sleep. And if all of that isn't bad enough, sleep deprivation totally kills your sex drive. So not fun!

So, obviously, sleep is job number one for models and for *you!* Here's what you need to know to get your slumber on and master your beauty sleep.

Make Sleep Your New Healthy Habit

Once you make beauty sleep a healthy habit, it's almost effortless. All you have to do is lie down and close your eyes. It's *way* easier than sweating it out at the gym, and often more effective! But making beauty sleep a habit isn't easy for everyone. You would think that sleep, being a natural human need, would come totally naturally, but for many people it doesn't. That's why you have to make it a habit.

It's so easy to stay up too late. You get wrapped up in some TV series, especially when it's the finale. Your favorite old movie from when you were a kid comes on, just when you were thinking about hitting the pillow. You're reading a book and you can't put it down. You're playing a game on your iPhone and it's so addictive! And time flies when you're on Facebook.

But sleep is more important than all of those things, and you can do all of those things some other time, when you've had enough sleep. As I'll discuss in Chapter 10, it takes about 20 days to develop a new habit, as well as to lose one, so you can't expect to phase out late-night snacking or a TV habit overnight. Because the best stuff comes onto the home-shopping channels at night!

Think of the beauty-sleep key as your parents telling you: *Go to bed!* Kids hardly ever want to go to bed, but their parents make them! You can make yourself. Force it for 20 days, and suddenly, it will feel like you've been beauty-sleeping all your life.

But *how* do you make beauty sleep a habit? These are some model secrets for getting the ZZZs you need.

PrioritiZZZe Your ZZZs

From this moment on, your main concern is getting to bed on time. Not boys, not Twitter or Facebook, not clubbing, not the dirty dishes or the laundry. Your number one love and priority is now beauty sleep!

I fiercely protect and preserve my beauty-sleep schedule. I started to prioritize beauty sleep because I was losing it. I was losing it traveling on airplanes or adjusting to new time zones and new beds. I was losing it in loud model apartments, where you have several girls in one house and one (or more) of the girls has nothing to do, so she's up all night or out partying and comes back drunk, calls her family in Russia, and has the loudest conversation (which you can't understand anyway), just before stepping on your head on her way to the top bunk as your alarm goes off because it's time to wake up. (This actually happened!) I was losing it because I was stressed, anxious, excited, or all of the above about a casting, a go-see (when you meet the client so they can determine whether they want to see you for a casting), a job, or even just a visit to the agency, because I knew I was going to be judged, scrutinized, and picked apart, and I knew it was more or less all about my looks. The only thing I was certain of was that if I slept, I'd feel and look a lot better than if I didn't.

Vegas is not a city known for sleep, but when I was there— not once but *twice* in one week—for work, I was more concerned about hitting the sheets than strolling the Strip! The first trip—for the grand opening of the Versace boutique—was followed by an awesome after-party at one of the hottest clubs that was sure to be full of all the who's who and "cool" people in Vegas. As models, my crew and I were VIPs, but none of us actually went because we had a 7 A.M. flight, and two of us had two jobs apiece back in L.A. the next day. Did we want to go to the after-party? Of course we did! I really wanted to go! But I was self-aware enough to make sure beauty sleep took priority.

Sure, there are times when we break the rules (flexibility is necessary in order to balance), but those are occasions when we have enough good nights of beauty sleep logged in our beauty-sleep banks. The occasional indulgence is fine as long as beauty sleep is your priority most of the time.

SUPERMODEL **SAYS . . .**

I like to add sodium bicarbonate (baking soda) to my water before bed to fight off acidity from the coffee that I occasionally drink. At night, I always drink catnip tea to help me wind down.

— Stefanie Wood, superchef and model, represented by PhotoGenics

AccessoriZZZe Your ZZZs

Just like I never leave the house without my iPhone, I never go to beauty sleep without my earplugs or my eye mask. Before you grumble about how uncomfortable eye masks and earplugs are, let me say: I totally agree! I've gone through at least 20 eye masks and have tried nearly all the earplugs on the market! I now know which ones are the best.

A good eye mask needs to fit and lie gently on your face because you'll beauty-sleep terribly if it shifts or digs into your skin. My pick: the silk eye mask with lavender from Aroma Home. I also like Bucky's, which I buy at Whole Foods. It's lightweight and keeps out the light; plus, it comes in cute patterns. Mack's earplugs rock (get them at your local drugstore). They look and feel like wads of gum—but not as sticky—that you jam into your ear, and they are comfortable. They are the model's earplug of choice (and also the best-selling earplug in America!). Warning: Sometimes the earplugs get stuck in your hair and might leave a little residue. Hairstylists have often questioned me about this!

You're going to need to do your own research and figure out which brands and styles work best for you (much depends on the shape of your head and your beauty-sleep position). But you know what that means, don't you? *Shopping trip!* A perfect way to moder-cize! And as long as you are out shopping, look for new pillows and sheets that will make you feel the most like getting good shut-eye. And cute PJs! Unless you like to beauty-sleep in the nude, in which case, go for it!

You also need to set the stage for good rest and make sure your surroundings are in sync for beauty sleep. Other accessories can make you more comfortable. How's the temperature? Are you comfortable? Add a small fan if you want to bring the temp down, or pile on a soft, cozy blanket if you prefer to snooze in a toasty cocoon. Research shows that the optimal range for nodding off is between 60° and 68°F. Keeping the room in this zone can actually help lower your core body temperature, which signals *your* soon-to-be Supermodel YOU body that it's time for beauty sleep. When your core temperature is too high, sleep is more difficult. But re-member, do what works for you. This is general information, and you might be the exception.

RitualiZZZe Your ZZZs

The more regular your nighttime habits, the easier it will be to fall asleep. Your body recognizes your sleep cues and starts to wind down, so ritualiZZZing your ZZZs is one of the best ways to get into the habit of a sound and effective beauty sleep.

Let's go back to the Versace event I told you about in the previ-ous section. Once I returned to the hotel suite I shared with fellow models Bianca and Tara, we all plunged into our nightly bedtime rituals that would help us easily drift off. We all took off our make-up (or at least as much of the globs of waterproof everything that we could scrape off our faces) and brushed our teeth, and I show-ered, too, because there was no way I was waking up early to rinse off. I wanted to maximize my beauty sleep!

Then we all packed up and set aside our travel clothes before going to bed so we wouldn't have to do it in the morning. We checked into our flights, arranged our cars to the airport, mapped out where we had to be so we knew how much time we would need, and basically took care of anything that would have kept us awake thinking about it. This is a great idea to help you sleep if you tend to worry and fret about what you have to do the next day.

We also *all* turned our cell phones on silent, and then we went to bed, early enough to make sure we got sufficient beauty sleep! No sitting up all night talking. No lamenting about the party we were missing. Our minds were set on beauty-sleeping. We'd per-formed our pre-sleep rituals and prioritized our sleep, and the next day, we were ready to go. Sorry, cute boys looking for a booty call!

You probably have a regular daytime schedule, which most models do not. That's good news for you—you're ahead of the game! Take whatever time you need before bed to wrap up or plan ahead for all the little to-dos that might stress you out and inhibit your beauty sleep. You might not need to pack a suitcase at night, but you can do small tasks that might nag at you, like get your clothes together for the next day and prep the coffeemaker so all you have to do is press a button in the morning. And maybe make your to-do list for the next day so you don't have to lie awake wondering what you need to get done tomorrow. Then your atten-tion can shift into relaxation mode, and you can turn your brain toward the bed.

So now that you've showered, chosen your most flattering pair of jeans to wear tomorrow, and prepped the fruit you need for your breakfast smoothie, it's time to slip between the sheets. Wait! You have one more step. Your personal beauty-sleep ritual is what's going to tell your mind and body that it's time to shut down and snooze.

When you have a special ritual that you do every night right before you go to sleep, you trigger a biochemical and physical response in your body. The more you do something and follow it with sleep, the more you will associate that ritual with sleep.

Typical model sleep rituals are lighting candles, doing aromatherapy, taking baths, drinking herbal tea, stretching, taking the dog out for one last potty break, texting or calling significant others to tell them good night and sweet dreams (since we're so often on the road), and just working on relaxing.

Model Behavior

My model friend Natalia sets herself up for a good beauty sleep by unwinding with a mug of chamomile tea and a hot bath. Kerry makes sure not to nap during the day so she's primed for a good beauty sleep and in bed by 10 P.M. at the very latest. She'll also do some brief meditation beforehand to clear her mind.

My model friend Shira can't fall asleep unless she has rubbed an extra-thick lotion all over her hands and body and put a touch of Aquaphor on her lips. Cassie flips on a white-noise machine that helps her mind relax (sometimes she prefers oceans sounds) and does some light stretching before climbing under the covers. And don't laugh, but when my model friend Krista was working in Thailand, she picked up a unique sleep accessory: she taps a small gong three times and reads a favorite poem.

Personally, I love lavender oil sprinkled on my pillow, and I always light candles at night to get my body in sleep mode. Of course, extinguish them before you go to sleep—please don't start a fire!

These things are triggers that will start to create biochemical and physical reactions in your body, like Pavlov's drooling dogs! Triggers work for all kinds of behavioral changes, so use them if you have trouble sleeping. Your individual routine should be easy enough for you to complete religiously and also be one that helps you drift off—not keeps you up, like watching too much TV, listening to stimulating music, or drinking a cup of hot chocolate!

And speaking of TV and hot chocolate, let's talk about the things you *shouldn't* do because they are sleep robbers. It's time to muster up some self-awareness and target the habits that are compromising your sweet skinny-slumber. We'll do more of this when you modelize your beauty sleep in Chapter 9, but here's your list of things to avoid.

Avoid Caffeine and Other Sleep RobberZZZ

At least after a certain hour, like 2 or 3 P.M., nix the caffeine, especially if you are sensitive to it. Some people can drink coffee and still fall asleep, but guess what? There is no way those people are getting quality beauty sleep! It's not a shocker that caffeine is a stimulant. It increases your heart rate and prohibits deep and restful beauty sleep. (Sorry, Starbucks!) Models love their coffee in the morning only; and don't think that passing on coffee, tea, chocolate, and soda—or choosing decaf—in the evening means you're in the clear. Even decaf versions have some caffeine, and contrary to popular belief, green tea has caffeine! I learned that lesson the hard way when working in Japan. I was so freaking wired every night and couldn't figure out why. Then one of the local models pointed out I had been guzzling green tea to unwind before bed because it was billed as "caffeine-free," but green tea contains 24 to 40 grams of caffeine per cup (coffee has 95 to 200 grams). That was enough to keep me tossing and turning. Anyway, drinking a lot of anything will keep you from getting your eight hours of rest because you'll be up peeing all the time.

I once did a fashion show that was followed by a "fashion event"—just an excuse for a party. But the models were paid extra to hang out and mingle until 9 P.M. After rehearsal, makeup, hair, and the actual show, I had been there for like seven or eight hours, and by the time it got to be 7 or 8 P.M., I was hungry and tired, and I was probably mixing up both sensations and my self-awareness was waning.

All the models were longing to eat, but the food (just champagne and hors d'oeuvres) was for the guests, not for us. We became so desperately hungry (so *not* Supermodel YOU), and it didn't help that we were in skimpy outfits, so we were also freezing, which made us want to eat more (as I'll discuss in later chapters). I caved and sneaked one of the yummy, insanely calorie-loaded chocolate desserts being passed to the guests.

By the time I got home, it was 11, and I was so incredibly tired, but I couldn't fall asleep . . . WTH? I lay there going over whatever reasons there might be for still being awake: *Did I have caffeine too late, am I stressed, is there too much light or noise in my room, or what?* I've mentioned this before—the importance of asking yourself *WTH?* (or *WTF?* or *Why?*)—but I want to remind you because it's so important as you gain self-awareness. When I can't sleep, I do it; when I'm stressed, I do it; when I'm overeating, I do it; and when I don't have enough energy to modercize, I do it. WTH? What happened to cause this imbalance in me? Asking and answering this question creates the mind-body connection that is personal to *you,* and if you examine what you've been doing closely enough, chances are you will recognize an imbalance in at least one of the Five Keys.

SUPERMODEL **SAYS . . .**

I only drink coffee on the days I'm working, and only before 10 A.M. I'm very sensitive to caffeine and it keeps me up late, so I try not to drink it regularly. It doesn't feel healthy to me!

— Brooke Ritchie, model and co-creator of Supermodeled
(www.supermodeled.com)

I couldn't think of anything until I remembered that yummy chocolate treat I had around 8 P.M. I would bet anyone that the cake had espresso in it. Later, I asked Cory Martin, the owner of the catering company that handled that event (and most of the big fashion events), and he confirmed it: "One of our most popular tray-passed dessert items is our 100 percent organic chocolate espresso truffle sweetened with natural agave. Even the most diet-conscientious guests can't say no."

Aha moment! Not only does chocolate contain a substance called *theobromine* that mimics caffeine, but that espresso kept me up all night! Score another point for self-awareness. Now I know to avoid those things—at least after noon.

More forbidden foods before bed:

— Anything sugary will raise your blood-sugar levels and keep you awake. Shooting in Morocco, I was obsessed with the Moroccan mint tea. They give it to you everywhere, and it's so yummy. I practically lived off it while I was there, but I didn't sleep a wink because the tea is both sugary and caffeinated! (I didn't find out about the caffeine until later—I thought it was herbal tea!)

— Alcohol might make you drowsy, but you'll have a horrible night's sleep. When the sedative effects wear off, you're left fidgety, your body temp fluctuates, and you're dehydrated. You're also more likely to snore.

— Fatty foods mean your body will work hard to digest them, and spicy foods lead to heartburn (you'll be up looking for the antacid pills).

Model Behavior

Sex might seem like a sleep enhancer, but it's actually a sleep robber—at least, for women. A Spanish study from the Sleep Disorders Unit of the Catalonia General Hospital revealed that sex relaxes men so they fall right to sleep, but it's likelier to make women feel more energized and awake. So as much as sex is good for you (it's modercize!), when you really need your beauty sleep, you might be better off getting your love on in the morning.

Don't Keep "Up" (Late at Night!) with the KardashianZZZ

Most models love to watch TV—*Glee, Jersey Shore* reruns, *Gossip Girl, Keeping Up with the Kardashians*. You might hate to miss an episode, but you should almost always choose beauty sleep over seeing how many "grenades" The Situation brought home. Dr. Hairston told me one of the biggest reasons people are wide-awake when they should be getting shut-eye is that they feel they can't miss "their shows." Her advice? Be thoughtful: Do you really like the show? Why? Will your world crumble if you use your DVR or computer and watch it at a more reasonable hour tomorrow instead of *right now?* And is it really, truly worth the price you will pay the next day?

Dr. Hairston suggests watching TV with purpose—kind of the way models eat. Remember, we make a point not to eat just because food is there. Instead, we consume what we need when we need it, or if we just feel like a taste. It's the same with your TV schedule. Avoid aimlessly flipping channels, and make a conscious effort to watch only the shows that you really care about. If you're just trying to zone out, do something else, like listen to music, read a book, or meditate. "Think about quitting your sleep-depriving activities like someone trying to stop smoking," says Dr. Hairston. If TV is your drug of choice, choose your ten must-see shows and start to slowly cut back until you only have one or two.

Drop the DoritoZZZ!

I'll bet when you're zoning out in front of the tube, you're also eating aimlessly. And when you focus on the latest fashion disaster on *Project Runway,* you're not paying any attention to the fact that you just downed an entire bag of Cool Ranch Doritos or chocolate-covered raisins. Self-awareness! Hello! These things are fine in moderation, but the fat in the chips or the caffeine and sugar in the chocolate are going to lead to fragmented beauty sleep. Actually, eating anything at all less than an hour before bed can interrupt your snooze time—even a salad (yeah, like you're eating salad during *Dancing with the Stars*). Instead of your body feeling relaxed and primed to drift off, it now needs to expend energy to digest the food you just ate.

"The moment you put something in your mouth when your body is trying to slow down and get some rest, it's screaming back at you: What are ya doing? It's time for bed!" says Dr. Michael Breus, aka "The Sleep Doctor" (**www.sleepdoctor.com**). If you do need a snack, opt for complex carbs and a little protein (like a slice of wheat toast with peanut butter), which is easier to digest than a pint of ice cream. Even just fruit at night can be a poor choice if you're sensitive to sugar, because fruit has a lot of sugar, even if it's natural.

Nerd Alert!

Another reason not to go on a crazy food binge before bed: the crap you eat right before you sleep is going straight to your fat cells, because you don't need energy when you're sleeping. Isn't it obvious? Researchers from Northwestern University found that eating late at night leads to more than twice as much weight gain as when the same foods are consumed during the day when you need them. "Eating at night is contradicting your body's natural circadian rhythm," the study's lead author, Deanna Arble, Ph.D., wrote. "Leptin levels are starting to rise, and are supposed to be discouraging you from eating." But instead, you're encouraging your body to chow down, and it gets confused and you end up gaining weight. When eaten at appropriate times, all of those calories would be turned into energy, not stored as fat. Eat during the day when you need the energy, not when you need your beauty sleep.

Hit the PillowZZZ, Not the Gym

A lot of models would rather modercize (Key 4) than sweat it out at the gym, and modercizing translates to "moderate exercise" by most standards. Studies have shown that moderate exercise in general can help you beauty-sleep better and longer at night. But don't hit the gym right before it's time for bed or your body will be too revved up for beauty sleep. Working out raises your body temperature, which is supposed to dip slightly at night, signaling your brain that it's time to calm down and start dreaming.

So even though you may have showered off all that sweat from your P.M. Zumba class or that moonlit game of beach volleyball, your body doesn't have the chance to cool down and go into beauty-sleep mode.

That said, I do have to admit that it's easy to talk me into a game of moonlit beach volleyball! Some friends and I actually played glow-in-the-dark volleyball one night! We painted the ball with glow-in-the-dark paint. But when the ball started losing its light charge, I realized this game could be dangerous— I was shooting in the morning, and getting smacked in the face with the ball probably wouldn't be a good idea. Self-awareness! So, I volunteered to be the "ball light charger." Basically, I held the flashlight up to the balls to activate the glow in the dark. It was fun! Sometimes, fun wins out over sleep—enjoying life is one of the best ways to embrace Supermodel YOU! But most of the time, sleep should score the winning spike.

Model Behavior

Supermodel Late-Night Turn-ons:	Supermodel Late-Night Turn-offs:
Relaxing music	Bright lights
Candles	Sex
Warm baths	Television
Hot herbal tea	Caffeine
Sleep masks	Junk food
Meditation	
Sexy massages	

Do Not Hit SnooZZZe

Many models need alarm clocks to wake up, but most don't bother with the snooze button. Instead, we set our iPhones to go off at the latest possible time in the morning. Do you hit snooze a million times? Lots of people do, but it's totally counterproductive and cuts into your beauty sleep. Once you hear that annoying buzz, your mind is jolted awake. Even if you can coerce your rattled self back to bed, your sleep is now fragmented, and it won't be as productive or beauty-beneficial anymore. Wouldn't it have been better if you had just peacefully slept a little later? In fact, you won't need the snooze button if you just go to bed early enough (like models do) so that you get seven or eight hours of rest! You *snooze* (button), you *lose* (as in you gain weight and lose your Supermodel YOU body!).

Model Pretty

Models rarely do their hair or makeup when they're not working. And you will probably never catch a model in the A.M. looking polished unless she's coming straight off a job. The reason: forgoing an elaborate beauty routine in the morning means we get more shut-eye (so we're naturally more beautiful!). Not that we want to look frumpy in public— and neither do you. But you don't have to, with model-pretty tricks. Put away your flatiron and set your alarm clock for an extra half hour (at least) of sleep time! Here are some quick model-approved tips for sleeping in but still looking pretty, chic, and fashionable:

- I have go-to outfits I don't even have to think about. I already know they are fashionable and comfortable.

- Unless you have a major date or a big presentation at work, you don't need a pile of makeup. Pare down your routine to the basics so you look polished in a minimal amount of time: under-eye concealer, a swipe of eye shadow, mascara, and some color on your cheeks. If you're just out shopping for the day or meeting friends for cappuccinos, skip the makeup and throw on some dark sunglasses (the bigger the better). You'll look instantly fashionable. If you pinch your cheeks and bite your lip (not too hard!), you'll get that rosy glow and rosy lips without any makeup at all.

- Hydration is huge, and a spritz of mineral water always makes your skin look prettier.

- Tinted sunscreen is an easy swap for makeup.

- Your hair is beautiful! You probably don't think so, which is why you spend waaaay too much time fussing with it when you could be asleep. Play with hair bands, pretty clips, and sleek ponytails for quick fixes. When models wake up with crazy hair (it does happen!), a hat or a hoodie can look supercute while taming your tresses.

- A good accessory or piece of jewelry makes you look pulled together.

- Good posture is the ultimate beautifier! It always makes you look prettier and more alert.

Oops, I Did It Again!: No Beauty Sleep = One KlutZZZy Model

I used to be a total klutz. A total *tired* klutz. But it wasn't just me. Models have to walk in ridiculously high shoes in shows, but nearly all of those embarrassing runway trips and slips can be attributed to lack of beauty sleep rather than the crazy footwear! Almost every major model has biffed it on the runway, and I can guarantee a lot of that has to do with not getting enough rest. You'll be forgiven if it happens once or twice, but eating it on the runway is not the best way to look professional: if we keep messing up, we're out of work.

I'm pretty sure I decided I was naturally clumsy in college when I wasn't sleeping at all. I was working a full-time job, going to school full-time, having a full-time social life, and working out like a maniac. There was *no* time to get shut-eye—or so I thought. I'd be walking down the street, and for no reason, stumble over my own feet! I always used to bump into things and get bruises. It wasn't until after finishing college and actually sleeping again, right before I started modeling, that I no longer found myself tripping over my feet and bumping into walls and counters I somehow failed to see.

I finally made the sleep-clumsiness connection during my first sleep-deprived fashion week in Milan. Halfway through the shows, I turned totally clumsy again. Even though I had only been modeling a few months and this was my very first fashion season, I knew tripping over my feet was *not* due to natural clumsiness or inexperience. It was due to lack of beauty sleep! Lightbulb moment! I realized that if I didn't start getting more sleep, I was going to fall flat on the runway and embarrass myself beyond belief!

Beauty sleep became my antidote—not only for clumsiness, but for all the other negative side effects of inadequate rest. Beauty-sleep deprivation was causing me a lack of energy, moodiness, poor concentration, depression, and negative thinking.

"Most people will show serious impairments if they are deprived of sleep for even a few days," says Dr. David Dinges, a sleep researcher at the University of Pennsylvania. "The problem is most people assume they are well rested when they are not." Thanks, Dr. Dinges. You just proved my point. When you're exhausted, you don't even have the self-awareness to realize you need sleep. You just think you can push through and maybe down an extra skim latte in the afternoon to keep you alert. Or, like me, you just label yourself a klutz who drops a lot of dishes, or a forgetful girl who is always losing her house keys, and leave it at that.

But since models are very self-aware about beauty sleep, we can shed most of the negative personality traits that all of the other exhausted people exhibit! Sure, there are plenty of times I don't get a good night's rest—when I'm working and my shoot runs into the late hours of the evening. It's beyond my control, but I am self-aware enough to be able to do some damage control and not let my overtired body and mind go haywire. And no more skidding out on the runway! (It happens to models every so often, and most falls are due to sleep deprivation and total exhaustion, although some incidents are due to getting caught in the dress, walking on a slippery runway, or other things totally out of your control—it's a dangerous job!)

■ ■

Now that you understand how important beauty sleep is for your body, your looks, your health, and everything else, it's time to make it a serious focus. Commit to sleep like you'd commit to Prince Charming! You won't believe how much prettier you'll look, how much better you'll feel, and how much easier it will be to lose weight and keep moving toward the body and life of your dreams. And when you get there, you'll want to be wide-awake so you can appreciate it all!

■ ■ ■

CHAPTER SIX

Key 3: De-stressing

This is a tough business. The pressures are enormous. If you want to succeed, you've got to stay creative and beat the stress.

— NICHOLAI FISCHER, SUPER–MOVIE DIRECTOR AND FASHION
PHOTOGRAPHER

Have you ever looked at yourself in the mirror when you're stressed? Try it next time. Do you have those little lines between your eyebrows because you're holding tension in your forehead? Do your eyes look a little frantic? Are the corners of your mouth turned down? And how do you feel? Is your heart beating faster? Do you want to punch something? Do you feel compelled to eat a cheesecake? Or do you want to just give up and crawl into bed?

For most of us, stress isn't pretty.

Some stress is good. We experience it for a reason. You get a rush like going on a roller coaster, and it can prime you to act quickly in an emergency. But chronic stress is totally different. Your body isn't meant to feel stressed all the time. That's so wrong. You can't live your life feeling like you might, at any second, have to run from a grizzly bear or save your whole family from a burning building. When you actually have to do those things, stress is awesome. It kicks your butt and puts you into superhero mode. But when those things are not on your to-do list, when you're just trying to work and make good food choices and enjoy your life, stress is a beauty killer, body destroyer, and home wrecker.

The American Institute of Stress estimates that 75 to 90 per-cent of doctor visits are related to problems caused by stress. Stress can make you sick, fat, and ugly because it causes you to lose sight of the other keys. It compromises self-awareness because your mind is too occupied with the subject of your stress. It ruins your sleep, which makes the stress even worse, creating a vicious cycle. It makes you eat when you don't really need or want to eat, causing unnecessary weight gain. It also makes you *less likely* to exercise. Good-bye, slammin' body! The very things that cause stress, like money problems and relationship issues, usually get a lot worse with chronic stress. Stress can cause road rage, violence, even suicide. Stress aggravates hypertension, insomnia, diabetes, herpes, and autoimmune diseases like multiple sclerosis. There's no question that stress hurts you physically, mentally, and emo-tionally. Living with chronic stress is one surefire way to stymie your inner supermodel.

But don't think for a minute that models don't have stress. Actually, it's the opposite. We have tons of stress. Modeling is one of the most stressful jobs. It may look easy. We just stand around looking pretty, right? No way! We have just as much stress as you do, even though the nature of the stress might be a little different.

But models can't afford to give in to the damaging effects of stress, like overeating, weight gain, bad skin, insomnia, and health problems, not to mention a frazzled brain that loses car keys or plane tickets or forgets what time to go to a job. We can't let stress take over our lives.

And neither can you, so let's start busting your stress, supermodel-style.

Financial Stress

Unless you were born rich, you probably know what it's like to experience financial insecurity. It can take a toll on your body and on your life. According to some of the sources I've seen, more than half of all divorces are caused by money problems. Being uncom-fortable financially is extremely stressful, and having to worry about how you're going to pay your bills can lead to unhappiness, poor relationships, weight gain, and a lot of other unhealthy side effects.

My model friend Natalia called me recently because she started gaining weight and couldn't figure out why. "I haven't changed anything!" she exclaimed. "I don't get it!"

"Are you sleeping?" I asked.

"Not really," she admitted.

Natalia had always been good about getting her eight hours of beauty sleep every night, but for the past few months she had been sleeping terribly, barely shutting her eyes for five hours a night! Why? She was stressed because she didn't have enough money to pay her bills.

Financial worries are the number one cause of stress in America, according to many different surveys I've seen. When you can't pay your bills, you live in fear of losing your basic security in life: shelter, warmth, food. When you have to worry that you can't pay for these things, your body goes into stress overdrive.

Models know this feeling very well. For one thing, models have zero job security. Almost every model, even the superfamous ones who don't have to be concerned about money now, has had to struggle with financial stress in the past. Yes, even Kate Moss and Gisele! Being a model is one of the most financially insecure professions out there! We are considered self-employed, and our agencies, which typically take 20 percent of anything we make, are like employment agencies that get us jobs.

The modeling industry is notorious for being a financially insecure employer. One day, you might make $7,000 shooting for some high-end catalog, and then not work again all year. We also have to worry about age, because with every passing year, we get older, and we have to do everything we can to stay looking young so we can keep getting jobs. All of this can make models feel extremely uncomfortable and completely stressed. No wonder we know so many beauty secrets—it's about survival!

Another one of the biggest financially stressful things is getting paid. Models don't get a paycheck until the client pays the agency. Then the agency takes their cut, and then they pay the model. Sometimes, it can take years to get paid, and sometimes you never get paid at all. I once did a job in Jamaica, and I don't remember what happened, but the client never paid and filed for bankruptcy or something, so I never saw a dime—and the job actually ended up costing me money because I had to pay my travel expenses. Awesome, right? Waiting to get paid is superstressful because, like everyone else, we've got bills, too!

Money stress not only makes you feel insecure, but can lead to depression, and that can make you totally forget the other keys. And stress can kill a modeling career, so we have to learn to deal with it. That's why models are so frugal when they buy clothes and cars, and why they are more likely to bring their own food than waste money on expensive restaurants.

Money stress gets to me, too, and it was especially hard when I first started modeling. Even though I'm in a better place now, the stress can still creep in, especially when I'm paying bills, so I've got a routine that works for me. Whenever I have to pay bills, I always say this affirmation: "I *love* paying my bills, because it means I have money to pay them!" It cracks me up to do this, but it works! Love your stress! Of course you hate it, but when you turn hate to love, magic happens. Love your stress, knowing that you created it and you can un-create it. Know that it's just your body doing what it thinks it's supposed to do to keep you safe from harm.

Job Stress

Most people have work-related stress, whether it's a deadline, a lame boss, too much on our plate, long hours, safety issues, job insecurity (which leads to financial stress), or just unpredictability. Studies show that people who never know what to expect at work have a lot more stress than people with a regular routine, and nobody knows that like a model.

For one thing, we work crazy hours. We're always getting yelled at, poked, and treated like subhumans. Maybe the photographer, stylist, or designer is yelling at us because we're taking too long to get our next outfit on, or because we don't want to cram our feet into size-7 shoes when we wear a 10, or because how dare we need to pee! We are often told we're not good enough.

Our jobs are so demanding that we struggle to stay in touch with friends and family, we rarely have enough time in the day to get everything done, and we rack up big bills but never seem to earn enough money to pay them. Because of our unpredictable schedules and the crazy jobs we have to do, we often end up having to break up with boyfriends (or they break up with us and find someone "steadier"), and we fight with our families because we can't be at family events or because we don't keep in touch often enough. Then, for our trouble, we wake up with monster zits on our faces right before one of the most important shoots in our career. This totally happened to me in Paris right before shooting beauty for *German Vogue* with fashion photographer Javier Vallhonrat, who is kind of a big deal! I felt so ugly. (Luckily for me, this guy can make anybody look beautiful. He's a supergenius!)

Our jobs are also physically stressful. For example, to save money, many clients will try to shoot too much in one day. One time, I think we shot 152 looks in one day. That means that we shot 152 different outfits, so I had to change clothes 152 times and come up with 152 different poses or positions that would best accentuate the clothes, times however many poses it took for me to nail the shot. I literally had no time to even go to the bathroom. It was hours of change, change, pose, pose, pose, change, change, touch up hair, touch up lips, change, pose, change, pose . . . by the end of day, I was exhausted. All that changing of clothes and posing burns major calories. Who needs the gym? I felt like I was changing clothes and posing at the same rate that a hummingbird flaps her wings!

FashionSpeak

A *look* is an outfit a model wears in a photo shoot or a show.

Then there are the times we don't get to move at all, and that can drive a fidgety model crazy! I once sat for five hours to have my hair done for a shoot. We spend a lot of time just waiting around while everybody else is getting ready, not to mention all the time we spend sitting on airplanes.

Another kind of physical stress involves how much models are touched, prodded, and arranged all day. The first time I had hair extensions put in, the stylist chopped my hair off in different lengths. *My hair!* She said she was only cutting the extensions and not my hair, but I could *see* her cutting it! She either lied or really messed up the job. I was devastated, but I didn't say anything because I had just started modeling and I didn't want to complain. After the shoot I spent hours ripping my hair out because I couldn't get the extensions off, and I think the stylist must have known she did something wrong because she didn't stick around to tell me how to take them out of my hair. I was crying. I was exhausted. It was 3 A.M. when I finally finished, and the stress was overwhelming.

Whatever your profession is, I know you have your own kind of job stress, so start thinking about what it is. In Chapter 9, I'll help you figure out what to do about it.

Travel Stress

Models travel a lot more than most people with more "normal" jobs, and the way we travel is extremely stressful because we never know when we're going to have to hit the road with barely a moment's notice. We literally get our schedules the night before. Sometimes, we'll get a heads-up, but we never know for sure until we get the actual call sheet, which comes from the agent once he or she receives it from the client. This is usually last-minute. Basically, if a client thinks they want to work with a model, they'll call the agent and see if the model is available, and they'll ask to either hold or option the model. A client will often option or hold more than one girl, because there are so many people who have to make the final decision and it's based on so many factors, including the model's rate, availability, the look, the fit, and so on.

Many times, you'll have more than one option for a given day, and this is when your agent will determine which client gets the first option or second option or third option. This is all based on who the client is, how much the job pays, and a bunch of other factors that I don't even know about, some of them likely pretty shady, like an agent telling a client you're available when you aren't, then pushing another model on them, or telling the client you aren't available even if you are, in order to push another model over you. I've heard horror stories about all of this, and I'm sure I've been an unwitting victim of it. But I digress—the point is that *we never know when we might have to travel halfway across the world at a moment's notice!* And that's stressful.

Sometimes I travel with other models. It's kind of fun and embarrassing at the same time. Like a herd of models doesn't get attention in airports! One time, the Southwest Airlines flight attendant announced over the intercom that runway models were on board. It was funny, but also mortifying.

You might think that all this travel sounds exciting, and sometimes it is when we get to go to a cool place, but even when it's exciting, it's also stressful. In order to not get completely overwhelmed and exhausted by this constant flux and travel, a model has to learn how to cope with this continual state of the unknown. And forget commitments. We can't commit to anything because we never know if we're going to be able to be there. Dinner tomorrow? Who knows! Our lives are full of winging it because we don't even know from one day to the next whether we'll be in town.

You might think: *Exciting! I'm off to Bangkok tomorrow!* We think: *Bangkok? Tomorrow? OMG! OMG! Okay, breathe! Gotta pack, gotta pack! What's the weather like there? What do I need? Where am I going afterward? Has my passport expired? Where is my friggin' passport?*

After Bangkok, we might end up flying to Antarctica or Cancún, so we pretty much have to be prepared for anything. It's very stressful to plan for the unplanned, so in order to avoid getting completely overwhelmed and exhausted by this constant on-the-go, we've developed a number of tricks to keep calm. Here are some of my favorite supermodel travel tips:

— **Check the weather.** Keep a weather app on your smartphone with the weather for your destination. Don't just assume because you're going to Hawaii that it's going to be tropical conditions. You never know if a storm is going to come or what. I once had a shoot in Ibiza, so of course I packed bikinis, short shorts, and little dresses. OMG! Let me tell you. It was so freezing cold. It was raining. It was windy. I thought I was going to die!

SUPERMODEL **PLAYLIST**

I'm always commuting from castings in Los Angeles to my house in Newport Beach, so I have a playlist titled "Traffic." It's calming, de-stressing, and yet passionate.

Coldplay, "Warning Sign"
Kings of Leon, "Knocked Up"
Moby, "Wait for Me"
David Guetta ft. Sia, "Titanium"
Sneaker Pimps, "6 Underground"
Slightly Stoopid, "Closer to the Sun"
Pretty Lights, "Finally Moving"
Broken Bells, "The High Road"

— Natalie Pack, gorgeous fashion model, Miss California USA 2012, and pre-med student at the University of California–Irvine

---

— **Pay attention to the time.** Know your flight times. Know when you have to leave. Have your ride/driver/cab pre-booked and be ready ahead of time. Check in the night/day before and print out your boarding pass. Have your travel documents ready, and don't forget your ID or passport! Even if I'm not planning to leave the country, I will always throw my passport in my suitcase in the event I lose my ID, and because it's so easy to switch purses and forget to switch my ID! (And besides, you never know when you might get a job booked in another country!) I also plan my travel time. If I'm flying a red-eye or just need some time to relax, I plan on that. If it's work time, I plan on catching up on my e-mails or book work. If it's entertainment time, I make sure I've downloaded movies onto my laptop.

— **Pack smart.** Shoes are heavy, so try to plan as many outfits as you can with the same pair of shoes while still looking cute and stylish, and wear your heaviest shoes on the plane. I like to modercize, so I always pack my gym shoes and gym clothes. I find that even if I don't have access to a gym or time to exercise (meaning time to move in whatever way feels good), just putting on these clothes inspires me to move more. Workout shoes and clothes take up more suitcase space, but they're totally worth it. If I'm going somewhere for an event, such as a wedding, I make sure to pack that stuff first, like the bridesmaid dress. Or if it's really heavy or cumbersome, I will ship it beforehand. I just did this with a Versace dress I had to wear for a charity event. That thing was gorgeous, but it weighed ten pounds, and besides, I didn't want to lose it! If you're traveling for an interview or another important event, pack the related stuff first, like your good suit. Then fit the fun clothes around those items. Also, remember to always have a cocktail dress, a swimsuit, and mix-and-match clothes so you don't have to pack an entirely new outfit for every day of your trip.

— **Go with what you know.** Never pack only new clothes or clothes you've barely worn. People like to go shopping for new clothes before they travel (I'm guilty), but too often, you put something on and realize it's not comfortable, or it doesn't feel right or look as good as you thought it did, and then you're stuck with nothing to wear. Stick with what you know is comfortable and works. Remember to follow the Supermodel Comfort Credo: *comfort first!*

— **Divide and conquer: carry-on vs. checked.** Check your clothes and shoes, but always have warm clothes and comfortable shoes with you for the travel part, and one change of clothes, a toothbrush, and personal-care stuff in your carry-on in case you get stranded overnight without your luggage.

— **Prepare to modercize.** Traveling is not glamorous. You can walk miles in airports or stand for hours in security lines, so be prepared for that. You want your travel experience to be enjoyable, so stay in shape and get used to a lot of walking and standing before you go. And remember to count that as exercise!

— **Bundle up, even in summer.** I always have a jacket or sweater or something warm. Flights are often freezing! They blast the AC in airplanes. Someone told me that the colder the air, the lighter the plane. I don't know if it's true, but they must keep it freezing for some reason! I always wear or bring socks for cold feet, and once the plane is off the ground, I take my shoes off and get comfy. They rarely give out blankets anymore, especially in coach (yes, models totally fly coach!), so make sure you have something to stay warm or get cozy with. A lot of models carry nice pashminas because they keep you warm and they're fashionable. Cashmere pashminas are heaven! Don't rely on the airline to provide something. You might get a skimpy little square of cheap flannel in a plastic bag. A pashmina is much more relaxing.

— **Stash your snacks.** I always keep snacks in my carry-on. It's my portable snack bar. Pack your own food, and pass on the plane food and "free" snacks and drinks, which are full of extra calories you probably don't need. Protein bars, fruit, baby carrots, nuts, water (you have to buy this after going through security, of course, because we all know how dangerous water is!). I recommend drinking extra water when traveling, even if you have to pee a lot in that amazing little airplane restroom, because flying is dehydrating and that's not good for beautiful bodies and skin.

— **Stress-proof your carry-on.** My carry-on always contains:

- Toothbrush
- Lotion (because, as I said, traveling is dehydrating for skin)
- Hand sanitizer (so many germs while traveling!)
- Spritzer for my face (like lavender water or even Evian spray)

- Gum (to help my ears with cabin pressure)
- Earplugs (planes can be loud—crying babies, people talking too loudly, the flight attendants and pilots constantly on the intercoms, and the horrible engine noise on those small planes)
- Eye mask (if I want to sleep)
- Pillow (some people like to bring one . . . I used to, but realized it wasn't necessary for me)
- Headphones, smartphone, tablet, and/or laptop
- Book or magazine
- ChapStick (hydration again: many models swear by Aquaphor or Elizabeth Arden's Eight Hour Cream; I'm a natural girl, so it's Burt's Bees, Hempz, or something like that)

— **Get good luggage.** Good luggage is so important! I cannot emphasize enough how amazing spinner wheels are! They allow your luggage to roll in all directions. I also have a standard travel bag and a few cute ones, of course. My favorites are my Stella bag and my BCBG bag, because I can almost always fit everything I need into one of them.

— **Take travel music.** Everybody has their own preferences; different kinds of music keep travel stress-free for different people.

SUPERMODEL **PLAYLIST**

I find that music is very personal. Each song evokes a different memory and mood. My favorite artist is Bon Iver. I listened to him throughout my travels in Europe. Now, every time I listen to him, I recall my past adventures.

— Michel Pilon, model, represented by PhotoGenics

— **Pack vitamins and medication.** Some people just can't manage the stress of travel and take antianxiety pills or sleeping pills. I used to depend on them, but I don't like taking any medications or relying on anything, even if it's herbal. I want my body to work! When I have the Five Keys in check and balanced, I rarely go awry and thus no longer need them. But if you do, don't forget to pack them! Have a small pillbox for your carry-on. Some girls swear by Airborne and other vitamin elixirs to combat germs and getting sick. Whatever you need, have it on hand!

— **Stow some melatonin.** This supplement is superawesome for resetting your body clock after making time changes, which really helps with jet lag.

Relationship Stress

Relationships? What are those? Actually, sometimes I'm not sure which is worse—never having enough time to have a relationship or being in a stressful relationship. Bottom line: they're both extremely stressful!

Models are always traveling, so relationships are hard. We spend a lot of time alone. The crews and people we work with constantly change based on our job, so establishing any real connection is challenging. There can be jealousy and cattiness between models, even though many I've met are amazing people. My agents are like my family right now, but some of the ones I've had in the past were nothing like family (at least not like a nice family!)—they see you as a commodity.

Dating requires a lot of self-confidence for models, even though you might think it's easy for us. One of the problems is that the nature of our job involves taking sexy pictures, getting a lot of attention, changing clothes in front of people, sometimes shooting naked. That can really bother some of our potential romantic partners, and a lot of relationships have fallen apart because of those things. We're always encouraged not to bring along boyfriends to shoots or during travel, and even when it's allowed, it's not like we have much spare time to spend enjoying the location.

FashionSpeak

International models—which includes all supermodels—have multiple agents because wherever you go, you deal with agents who book your jobs. And when you travel to the lucrative markets in other countries (besides New York and Los Angeles, the lucrative markets are Milan, Paris, London, and Tokyo), you need agents in those cities.

A mother-agent is usually the agent or agency that found or discovered you. The mother-agent trumps all agencies. They basically sign a contract with you, and then sell you to other agencies and markets. They will make a commission off the commission that the other agencies take.

My career was launched in L.A. by PhotoGenics, so they are my mother-agent, but I was sent right away to an agency in New York, who then sent me to an agency in Paris, who sent me to an agency in Milan, and so on. If you pick up steam in one market, other agencies then want you, too. Sometimes, you don't have any idea who represents you, where. At one point, I had my mother-agent in L.A., and also agents in New York, Milan, Paris, London, Tokyo, Germany, Spain, and probably a few more places as well. Right now, I'm back to having agents only in the main markets: New York, Paris, Milan, Los Angeles, and Germany.

Health Stress

Stress can cause illness, and illness can definitely cause stress. If you have a health issue, you might worry about it a lot, and you might also just feel bad, which can make you slip up on all the other keys, which only makes stress worse. Models need to stay healthy by getting enough sleep, eating right, and moving our bodies.

We can't afford to get sick and miss a job or look all red-nosed or puffy, and I know *you* can't afford to get sick, either. When you do, it's important to follow the Five Keys so you can heal as quickly as possible. Practice the stress-reduction techniques at the end of this chapter every day if you can, but especially when you're sick or have a health issue.

I think we can all agree that chronic stress is worth reducing. Think about some of your most stressful moments and how drained they have left you. We all have some of the same stressors and some different ones, but the point is that if you don't deal with them properly, they will negatively affect your body and your health.

SUPERMODEL **PLAYLIST**

*These are songs for winding up and winding down! My taste in music changes by the week, but here are some songs I never get sick of (or haven't yet). A good place to find these and other songs is **www.hypem.com** or on my music blog, **www.fifthgiant.com**.*

The Units, "High Pressure Days" (Rory Phillips Remix)
Rebecca & Fiona, "Bullets" (Club Mix)
Soft Powers, "Ozymandias (Never Meant To)"
Metronomy, "The Look"
Purity Ring, "Ungirthed"
Yacht, "Psychic City (Voodoo City)"
Marina and the Diamonds, "Oh No!" (Grum Remix)
Robyn, "Dancing on My Own"
Foster the People, "Helena Beat"
Grimes, "Genesis"
Matthew Dear, "Soil to Seed"
Bot'Ox, "Blue Steel"
Father John Misty, "Hollywood Forever Cemetery Sings"
Best Coast, "Summer Mood"
Local Natives, "Wide Eyes"
Wild Nothing, "Chinatown"
Real Estate, "Out of Tune"
Perfume Genius, "Learning"
Phantogram, "Turn It Off"
Damien Jurado, "Rachel & Cali"

— Jenny Bahn, model and superawesome writer/blogger
(**www.jennyblovesyou.com**)

Model Secrets for Reducing Stress

Now how does a model deal with all of this stress? Here are a few tips for how my model friends and I handle some typical stressful situations.

— **Mellowing out with Mozart.** When I'm modeling in Los Angeles, I spend hours stuck in traffic. It's enough to make anybody crazy! The only way I can keep from getting totally stressed is by listening to classical music. Sorry, Lady Gaga! Love you, but Mozart does it for me when it comes to traffic. I also like audiobooks for long trips. You get somewhere, and the book transports you somewhere else at the same time!

— **Fashionably late?** Not models! Well, maybe we are . . . but we try not to be! Being late always used to be a huge source of stress in my life, so one day I decided to make being on time a serious priority. It's changed my life! I always plan ahead, so I allocate time for traffic, accidents, and other unplanned events. When you're running late, your body responds to that stress in exactly the same way as if you were running from a wild animal that wanted to eat you. Your body doesn't know the difference. So quit being late! Decide to stop. When I did this, it dramatically reduced the stress in my life.

I actually got this *Aha* moment about being on time from Ryan Seacrest. I was listening to his radio show, and he was talking about the keys to weight-loss success that his personal trainer taught him. This was one of them. I was like, *OMG! That's so me!*

On the show, they called being late "stupid stress" because it's something you do that you have complete control over, and it's destroying your body, yet you keep doing it. Duh! Research totally supports how being late is a chronic stressor. According to psychologist Linda Sapadin, Ph.D., author of *Master Your Fears,* when you are chronically late, "you're creating a reputation for yourself, and it's not the best reputation to be establishing. People feel they can't trust you or rely on you, so it impacts relationships. It also impacts self-esteem." Wow. If that's not a reason to lay out your clothes and make sure you've got your car keys located the night before, I don't know what is!

— **Jammin'.** Music is a giant magical stress reliever that models totally embrace! Music can invoke particular moods or states of mind. It can energize you, mellow you out, make you emotional, make you feel passionate, or help you fall asleep. Models often use music to chill-ax (like before a big show when we're anxious or nervous). We use it to motivate ourselves, we use it when we modercize—we use it for *everything!* Models are notorious for having their headphones on and the outside world tuned out, especially during long makeup or hair sessions or while walking through the city. When situations in our lives get stressful, we pop in our earphones. We also do it to avoid getting caught up in cattiness during casting. Models like to zone out to music so we don't get stressed out looking around and imagining what people are saying, or thinking too much about someone's negative comment. It's major therapy for us.

Because of its de-stressing effects, music can not only calm you but also help you fall asleep and even help you lose weight. If you feel a binge coming on, get totally immersed in some of your fave songs instead. Humming or singing along to music also helps me chill (and avoid mindless snacking). The music varies from model to model, but everyone knows what music can calm them, distract them, or get them pumped up. Make playlists according to the mood you need to evoke in yourself.

— **Reading.** Models have to spend a lot of time waiting, and despite the stereotypes, we totally love reading! Okay, sure, we're partial to fun books like the *Harry Potter* series, all the *Twilight* books, and *The Hunger Games* trilogy, but we also love nonfiction books, especially ones about health, fitness, and self-help. I think part of the reason why models love to read is that a lot of them didn't finish high school or didn't go to college. We have a lot to learn! So we educate ourselves on the subjects that interest us.

— **Meditating.** Maybe it sounds supercheesy or like hocus-pocus mumbo-jumbo to you, but meditation actually works. Studies have proved it. It lowers your blood pressure and clears stress hormones out of your body. Models employ some unique meditation techniques to manage stress. We aren't necessarily meditating according to some ancient esoteric tradition. When people think of meditation, they often think of monks and yoga rooms with people chanting and being all weird. When models meditate, it's more like we just close our eyes and go inward so we aren't distracted by what's going on around us.

Sometimes when the photographer gives me directions for what he or she wants for the shoot, I will meditate on that and get into that space, idea, or feeling. For example, if they say that they want me looking regal, I will meditate on being a queen while they're doing my hair and makeup. I pretty much meditate every time I'm in makeup and hair, which means I'm quiet and don't talk or engage in conversation with the makeup artist and hairdresser. I do this especially when I'm tired or stressed already and/or when I notice and pick up on their negative energy. I don't want to absorb it, so I go inside. That usually requires tuning out my senses and tuning in to some relaxing music and closing my eyes (even for a few seconds).

This model meditation (modeltation!) does wonders for relaxing out of the stress that comes from simply using your eyes all day. Vision is our strongest sense, so it uses most of our internal energy and also stresses us the most because we're constantly bombarded by images, pictures, and signs. Our eyes never get a break. We don't even realize how relaxing it can be to just let that go for a while. Try it! Just close your beautiful eyes for a few seconds and take a deep breath. This simple visual break can restore your sense of self, your feelings of sanity, even your beauty. It's just one form of meditation that allows all activity to settle down, and often results in the mind becoming more peaceful, calm, and focused. In essence, meditation rejuvenates your self-awareness. It restores clarity after a long, hard day of working and thinking.

You can try this in whatever you do that doesn't take your full attention. Don't do it while driving, of course, but you could meditate while on the subway, in line, waiting for a friend to pick you up, or traveling. Or just take some time to sit quietly and turn inward every morning or evening. Meditate on your beautiful self and you'll become more beautiful, because you'll be less stressed and more focused on what's important in your life.

SUPERMODEL **SAYS . . .**

Take time every day to meditate, weed out negative thoughts, and try to understand the root of negative thoughts. When you work on yourself mentally and spiritually (as well as physically), it will greatly improve your self-esteem.

— Marion Sealy, model, represented by PhotoGenics

— **Beauty breath.** One of the body's involuntary processes could be the simplest way to relax if you do it right. Being able to take a deep breath releases tension so it doesn't build up and turn into stress lines on your face. It relaxes you, fills you with energy, and makes you feel better. The end result: you look prettier! Whenever I'm feeling stressed or need to get focused, I take a long, deep beauty breath and I come back to myself.

I like to make triggers to help me remember my healthy habits, and beauty breathing is one of the things I always want to remember to do. When I have a wind fan on me for shoots to blow my hair back and move my clothes, it makes me really cold, but I use that as a trigger to remind me to breathe deeply. Think about things that could trigger your deep-breathing awareness, like every time you hear a siren or a certain song or a car horn honking. The more often you remember to breathe deeply, the less stressed you will feel almost immediately.

MODEL **TALK**

I use wind machines on studio shoots a lot because I love the way wind plays in the hair, giving the picture a sense of freedom, movement, and the great outdoors.

— Andrew Macpherson, superamazing fashion
and celebrity photographer

— **Focusing on the positive.** Another thing a lot of models do to relieve stress is to look at pictures of family, friends, and fun times they've had. Something about seeing those pictures, especially for visually oriented people, really helps make you feel calm and happy.

—**Talking.** Even though models spend a lot of time alone, or with an ever-changing entourage of agents, makeup people, hairdressers, and other models, we often find people to talk to—even the person sitting next to us on the airplane. That's when we vent, and we often get really good advice because the people we talk to don't know us that well, so they can be more objective. Try it!

— **Modercizing.** You'll read more about modercizing in the next chapter, but this model form of exercise is important for stress relief. Actually, *all* forms of exercise are good for stress relief. Exercise is the one method of stress relief that works for everyone. All you need is 30 to 40 minutes of moderate cardiovascular exercise like brisk walking, running, dancing, riding a bike, playing with kids in the park . . . even shopping! (But don't let stress trick you into spending more than you should, or you'll just be back to more financial stress!)

The bottom line is that stress is simply a part of life, but it doesn't have to take over your life. To access your inner supermodel, you're going to have to get a handle on it, and every part of your life will benefit when you do. So take a deep breath, turn up the volume on your iPod, and go for a walk. Keep your head up and walk with confidence, letting your mind disconnect from your stress, and you'll start feeling like Supermodel YOU again.

■ ■ ■

CHAPTER SEVEN

Key 4: Modercizing

The four biological pillars that contribute to well-being are: nutrition, sleep, exercise, and relaxation. . . . After exercising, your body may feel pleasantly relaxed physically, while mentally sharp, focused, and clear.

— DR. GABRIELA CORA, SUPER–VICE CHAIR OF THE COUNCIL ON COMMUNICATIONS FOR THE AMERICAN PSYCHIATRIC ASSOCIATION

Gym? Who's Gym? Some guy I used to date?

Here's how you work out like a model: Put on your Lululemon or Juicy Couture or Bebe Sport workout outfit. Check yourself out in the mirror to see how cute you look. Now go out and do a little shopping or run some errands. Strut your hot body. And welcome to modercizing!

Models are *so* not interested in sweating it out on a treadmill, lifting weights, or doing any kind of boring exercise. We want to have fun! Okay, some models love running or doing yoga or spin classes (myself included!), but more often than not, they don't go to the gym, and they think working out is a total snoozefest. Boring! Unless we know for a fact (and have preferably seen photographic evidence via a text message) that there are a lot of hot guys at the gym, we're not interested. And even then, we'll probably just play around when we get there, strolling along on the treadmill while we scan the room for who's flirtworthy.

But that doesn't mean we aren't getting a workout. Models stay thin, not because they overexert themselves at the gym, but because they *modercize.*

As explained in Chapter 3, modercize is a model's version of exercise, which includes nontraditional exercise activities that nevertheless burn calories, such as dancing, cleaning, changing clothes multiple times during work, shopping, and even making out with your significant other (kissing burns calories!). One of the most common forms of modercizing is fidgeting: sitting in chairs all day for hair and makeup can turn even the most patient model into a notorious fidgeter because it's so hard to sit still for that long. Also, music and fashion shows go hand in hand, so when they play music backstage, it makes us want to move—we bop, bounce, dance—but because we're supposed to be sitting still, it becomes "fidgeting." But this is good (the person putting on our mascara may not agree!) because we end up burning tons of calories that way.

Incidental Exercise = Modercize!

Do you realize that you probably already get exercise every day and don't even know it? And since you're not aware of it (Key 1), neither is your body, and therefore you don't reap the benefits. So start tuning in to when you move, how you move, and opportunities to move that you might not be taking advantage of. For example, do you know how many calories you burn just by showering and getting dressed? The average person burns more than 100 calories by taking a shower, getting dressed, and prepping for the day, but if you do it to music, or with extra energy, you'll burn even more. That's like walking on a treadmill for 20 minutes!

According to a Harvard Medical School newsletter, you burn about 150 calories walking for half an hour, and if you pick up the pace, you could burn almost 200 calories. How do you do that? By *noticing*, and walking straighter, faster, and with more purpose. Everything you do burns calories, but the way you do it affects how much you burn. Just a few tweaks here and there to add movement to your day, and momentum to your movement, can add up to major calorie torching that will make a real difference in achieving your ideal body. Household chores are great calorie burners, too. Weeding burns about 140 calories in 30 minutes. Mowing the lawn burns about 165 calories, and shoveling snow burns 180. But you don't even have to exert yourself that much. Cooking burns 75 calories in half an hour, grocery shopping with a cart burns 105 calories, heavy cleaning burns 135 calories, and playing with kids burns about 150 calories. Even sleeping burns about 20 calories per 30 minutes.

I read this really cool study about fidgeting. For 24 hours, 177 test subjects stayed inside a 10-by-12-foot respiratory chamber that measured everything they burned. All the subjects slept, ate, and exercised on a stationary bike during their time in the chamber, and could move around as much as they wanted to. The crazy thing was that there were huge differences in the number of calories the various subjects burned during the 24 hours. Some burned only about 1,300 calories, while others burned 3,600 calories! That's a giant difference, even when the researchers adjusted for muscle mass, and they concluded that the only difference among the subjects was how much they fidgeted. The high burners paced, played cards, and moved around all the time, rather than just sitting or lying down.

MODEL **TALK**

Most people hit the gym regularly, but they succumb to long periods of inactivity during the rest of their day. This is asking for trouble.

— Dr. Joseph Mercola, super–alternative physician

Do you realize what that means? You could potentially lose one pound every ten days, or 36 pounds in a year, just by allowing rather than stifling natural movement!

The trick is to realize how many calories you are burning all the time, and to make that mind-body connection. It might seem like hocus-pocus, but it really works. Feel how much you're burning. Make an effort to move, shift in your seat, get up often, tap your foot, look around, play with your hair, grab your phone and text, pace, jump up and down when you get a burst of energy . . . whatever it takes. You can amp up your burn way beyond what you might think, just by being one of those people who can't sit still.

Isn't that so much easier than going to the gym? In fact, over-exerting yourself at the gym can actually have the reverse effect on your body and cause you to gain weight because (1) you're going to be a lot hungrier, and you're going to eat more; and (2) you could injure yourself, and then you might not even be able to modercize as effectively. Working out should never make you gain weight! What's the point, then? I'll bet you can think of a million things you'd rather do than go to a sweaty gym and stare at the little TV on the treadmill for 45 minutes. Wouldn't you rather go shopping, go to the park, or make out with your boyfriend? (Although if you're going to watch TV, it's better to do it on the elliptical trainer at the gym than while vegging out on the couch, as long as you're in moving-more mode!)

High-fashion models need to be thin and fit, not bulky and muscle-bound (fitness models need to have more muscles). We aren't competing in bodybuilding contests. We just want to look pretty in nice clothes. So unless you really need all those muscles for some reason, spare yourself the effort. Six-packs and big biceps look hotter on boys anyway.

The point is to move the way your body wants to move. For some models, that means regular running. For some, it means tons of yoga. For others, dancing, shopping, walking, and fidgeting are plenty of movement. It all depends on you and what your body needs to stay in energy balance.

SUPERMODEL **PLAYLIST**

While running through Central Park, I go about five miles, so I need a long playlist. I like to pick upbeat music to keep me motivated. I like to mix newer songs with some older favorites. Some of the songs I choose make me feel powerful or sexy (usually the ultimate goal for working out). But most importantly, every song I work out to makes me want to boogie. That makes working out so much more fun!

The Ting Tings, "That's Not My Name"
Rihanna, "Only Girl in the World"
Katy B, "Katy on a Mission"
Maroon 5 ft. Christina Aguilera, "Moves Like Jagger"
La Roux, "Bulletproof"
Katy Perry, "Part of Me"
Martin Solveig & Dragonette, "Hello"
David Guetta ft. Nicki Minaj, "Turn Me On"
Katy Perry, "Hot N Cold"
Jesse J, "Domino"
Bow Wow ft. Chris Brown, "Ain't Thinkin' 'Bout You"
Katy Perry ft. Kanye West, "E.T."
Christina Aguilera, "Prima Donna"
Rihanna, "Birthday Cake"
Beyoncé, "Crazy in Love"
Carly Rae Jepsen, "Call Me Maybe"
Rihanna, "Where Have You Been"
Justin Bieber, "Boyfriend"
Eve, "Tambourine"
Kanye West, "Stronger"
Lady Gaga, "Starstruck"
Paramore, "Misery Business"
Ciara ft. Ludacris, "Ride"
Lil' Kim, "The Jump Off"
Beyoncé ft. Shakira, "Beautiful Liar"

— Julie Henderson, supersexy *Sports Illustrated* supermodel

The Fun Theory

I recently saw the most amazing video on YouTube. It was based on an initiative by Volkswagen that tries to get people to move more by making movement fun. The video I saw was of a staircase next to an escalator in a subway in Stockholm, Sweden. Cameras installed over the area showed that almost everyone chose the escalator over the stairs. Then, designers installed a system on the stairs that made them look like piano keys, and when people stepped on the stairs, the keys played notes. Suddenly, the video changed—people were fascinated by the piano-key stairs. A few stepped on them and heard the music, and then almost everyone flocked to the stairs. People jumped on the steps, went up and down, and were having so much fun. Overall, 66 percent more people chose the stairs when the piano keys were in place. (Check it out at: **www.thefuntheory.com.**)

The point is that if movement is fun, then maybe you'll actually do it! But I want to take this a step further. Part of having modeltude is to just decide that movement *is* fun. That taking the stairs is more fun than standing on the escalator, that walking is more fun than riding in a cab, that dancing is more fun than sitting at a table in a club swilling beer. Fun! Have fun! This is what models do, and this is what you can do. Life is your playground, so play!

Posture Check

Am I really going to harass you about your posture again?! I have to, so you don't miss the opportunity to burn major calories just by standing, sitting, and walking like a supermodel. Practicing supermodel posture is one of the easiest ways to modercize. Models don't just slowly stroll around. They strut with confidence and purpose, and they're burning more calories than the girl who is leisurely wandering or whose body language says, "Don't look at me!" Let your body language shout, "I'm a supermodel!"

That means standing tall and confident whenever you're standing, whether it's at home doing the dishes or in line at the supermarket or at a model casting. Slumping or sinking into one hip with all your weight on one foot is *not* modercizing. Walking like you're always on the runway *is* modercizing. Practice every chance you get. Putting triggers in place to remind you to sit, stand, and walk like a supermodel can be a great way to get yourself into this habit. Here are some ideas:

- Every time you catch your reflection in a mirror or a pane of glass, activate your supermodel posture!

- Every time you're standing in any line, activate your supermodel posture!

- Every time you enter a room, activate your supermodel posture!

MODEL **TALK**

Aesthetically, pulling your shoulders back and standing up straight can make you appear 10 pounds slimmer and more confident.

— Ashley Conrad, superbadass celebrity and supermodel trainer

This is the mind-set I want you to remember, adopt, and personalize. When you make an entrance, when you always hold your body like you're someone everybody wants to know, then you become that person. Your body changes, your mind changes, *you* change. You will look better, feel better, burn more calories, and be healthier.

Remember, supermodels aren't born. They're made. They weren't always confident, with great posture and body language. They weren't always so self-aware and in control of their habits and food choices. All of that developed over time, out of necessity for their profession. All you have to do is decide that confident body language, great posture, and healthy habits are a necessity for *you*. Pretty soon, you'll be vacuuming like a supermodel, carrying a laundry basket with your core in, making an entrance when you go to the gas station, and turning heads at your kid's school conference (just don't embarrass her too much!). It's all a matter of what you decide to do and who you decide to be. And it all starts with how you hold your body. Pretty soon, you'll be a natural.

MODEL **TALK**

I don't exercise. If God had wanted me to bend over, he would have put diamonds on the floor.

— Joan Rivers, supercomedienne

Natural Exercise = Modercize

When exercise is natural, it becomes what the body wants to do, without you having to force it. When the other keys are balanced—when you are self-aware, sleeping enough, and managing your stress—your body will want to move, and you will just naturally move throughout your day. Even if you have a desk job, when you feel the urge to get up and walk around or stretch, do it! If you are listening to music, dance, jump around, act out the song ("Y-M-C-A . . . !"). Pay attention to your natural urges. That's self-awareness.

And think about how humans used to live before technology. We hunted, gathered, gardened, played, spent a lot of time outside, and walked or ran to where we needed to go (or maybe rode a horse). Now, everything is done for us, but modercizing also means saying no to some of that. Do you have to take the escalator when the stairs are right there? And if you take the escalator, can you at least *walk* up the escalator? OMG! This makes me crazy! People get on the escalator and they just stand there. They even stand on those moving-sidewalk things at airports—it's called a moving side-*walk!* And these are young people I'm talking about, not people who are older or have mobility problems. These are people who could easily walk, but don't, because we're programmed not to—we're programmed to move as little as possible, and that's so damaging for our health, beauty, and overall balance.

Do you have to drive to your mailbox? Do you have to lie on the couch when you're talking on the phone? Do you have to watch TV horizontally? Do you have to stay inside all the time?

Truthfully, most models can afford to be superlazy because we've already learned that to be in energy balance, we eat and exercise as much as our individual bodies need to. If we don't move as much, we just know to eat less. Avoiding the extra calories you don't need in the first place is far more effective for achieving your supermodel body than spending more than a half hour on the elliptical machine just to burn off the 300 calories from the chocolate cupcake you ate because you were bored.

And since models are so smart about this, they don't need to exercise to lose weight—it's enough simply to have fun, de-stress, be healthy, meet boys, look cute in gym clothes, appear athletic, and socialize. We burn *tons* of calories that way. You can, too.

SUPERMODEL **SAYS . . .**

Exercise decreases the stress hormones such as cortisol, and increases endorphins. When you exercise, your body also releases adrenaline, serotonin, and dopamine. These hormones work together to produce feelings of euphoria and a general state of well-being, so during and after exercise, your mood is boosted naturally.

— LoLo Menghia, model and Romanian track star

But my point isn't to tell you that you should or shouldn't exercise. What I want you to get from this is that when you are self-aware and tuned in to your body, rather than being driven by a lack of balance in the Five Keys, your body will naturally seek out its own balance. It will *want* to move when it *needs* to move, and when you are self-aware, you will perceive that, and then you'll say yes to that beach volleyball game or that walk in the park. You'll get off the couch because you *want* to get off the couch. You'll pace or fidget because you're bursting with energy! And your weight will normalize.

So at first, you may need to think more about modercizing, and push yourself a little to encourage the habit of natural movement and to get your weight back to where it's meant to be. But then, to keep itself in homeostasis, your body will seek out the amount of movement and the amount of food it needs. So even if you're still working toward your goal weight, if you're healthy and following the keys, your body will go the right way. Just remember: less movement means you'll need less food, and self-awareness will help you feel that. But if you love to eat, then love to move, too. Find your energy balance. Food is potential energy, and movement is how you expend that potential energy.

Modercizing!

One of my favorite outdoor activities is playing beach volleyball. It burns tons of calories and is a blast! My model friends are always down for a beach playday, and they suck at volleyball (most of them)! They just want to strut their *skealthy* little bodies around in swimsuits and meet other beach-body hotties! Plus, there's a bonus: sunlight stimulates your pineal gland, which releases serotonin and makes you happy and causes your appetite to decrease. This is probably part of the reason why people tend to gain weight in the winter and lose it in the summer!

And if you aren't into sports? No problem. Have fun watching. Jump around and cheer. Even walking on the sand is a workout! It's freaking hard! So while my model friends aren't getting as much activity as I am playing volleyball, they're definitely burning calories. It's all modercizing, and it's all fun!

Fidgety Models Are Skinny Models

I have to get back to this idea of fidgeting because it's such a model quality. Kids always want to move, and adults are always telling them to sit still and stop fidgeting. It's too bad, because fidgeting and movement are natural and healthy, and we get this instinct drilled out of us. But I say it's time to reclaim your natural tendency to fidget! Models do it all the time, and so can you.

When I was a kid in school, I was in the band and played the drums. I've always heard music in my head, and the drums were the perfect outlet for this. I then found myself constantly tapping my foot or strumming my fingers whenever I was sitting. I often got in trouble in class for making noise, but that didn't stop me. I still do it, and it makes me happy. I especially love when I see others jamming out on the steering wheels of their cars or jumping around playing their air guitars at a club. This is the natural movement we suppress—the pure joy of moving, jumping, dancing, and finding a beat in our bodies. It's time to let this out! Sitting still is *not* natural for humans. Neither is a gym or a machine, but moving is! We should encourage movement, bopping, walking, tapping, and the like—letting the movement out.

Modercizing!

Can Nicki Minaj help you get a supermodel body? Upbeat music actually makes you move more and move faster, burning even more calories than mellow music. Singing along to music also burns calories and prevents mindless eating. You can't sing "Super Bass" if you've got food in your mouth!

I think I'm every hairdresser and makeup artist's worst nightmare. I cannot sit still for more than 20 minutes to save my life! After that, I'm going out of my mind if I can't move. Makeup typically takes about an hour, and hair usually a little less, but sometimes it can take up to five hours! Once, in Paris, I sat still long enough for them to give me this crazy hairdo that weighed more than I did when we were finished, and boy, did I drive that hairdresser crazy! I also had to sit for three hours once in Tokyo, getting my nails done for *one photo* in *Vogue* that was highlighting the $100,000 Cartier ring on my finger.

So even though I might suggest that some models are lazy, I would never say we're sedentary. When we have to sit, we're bopping to our music, texting, or jabbering with the model next to us. Sometimes I wonder if most models have ADD! Having makeup done is actually fairly active and takes some concentration—not easy for me, or most models! We can't just relax and get pampered in the makeup chair like people might think, especially when they're doing our eyes and lips. It's constantly: "Look up, look down, look up and to the right, close your eyes, open your eyes, pucker your lips, don't pucker your lips, smile, don't smile." Ugh! Sometimes it makes me want to scream, "Leave me alone!" But of course, they're just doing their job.

Sometimes, makeup artists will tell me to look up, and I'll look up for like five seconds and then totally forget where I'm looking. Then they yell at me: "I said 'look *up*'!" They're probably thinking, *Stupid model! How hard is it to look up?* It's kind of hilarious.

My point is that I think of all this as modercize. Fidgeting is modercize! Every little movement you make can and does add up to calories burned. If you have a sedentary job, one of the best ways to entice fidgeting is music, so if there's any way at all to sneak it in, do it! But if you can't, even just remembering to adjust your weight is a lot more effective than not moving at all. Can you sit on one of those exercise balls as a chair? Can you tap your feet or your pencil? Rock back and forth a bit? You might annoy your cube mate, but you'll be burning calories. Make fidgeting a habit! And always remember your supermodel posture, even at your desk. Is your core in? Are your shoulders back? Is your head up? *Now* you're modercizing!

SUPERMODEL **PLAYLIST**

I love hip-hop such as gangsta rap when I'm working out! This is silly, but it gets me in the mood to run fast: I pretend the cops are chasing me! On Pandora I always use E-40 radio. He is this rapper I like from the Bay Area.

The Notorious B.I.G., "Hypnotize"
Wu Tang Clan, "C.R.E.A.M."

Kriss Kross, "Jump"
Ludacris ft. Lil Wayne, "Last of a Dying Breed"
David Banner, "Like a Pimp"
DMX, "Where Da Hood At"
Jay-Z, "On to the Next One"

— Janica de Guzman, supergoofball and superawesome model
who always makes me laugh, represented by L.A. Models Runway

How to Dress for Modercize

Models get to wear some of the most beautiful, extravagant, expensive clothes in the world. It's crazy what we have access to! I did a fashion show for De Beers where I wore a dress that was covered in diamonds. The dress was worth millions! To me, that's ridiculous—who would really wear that? If we actually wore jewel-encrusted gowns, six-inch stilettos, and body-hugging clothes in everyday life, we'd be packing on pounds because we can hardly move in those things!

Models dress for comfort, which, whether they know it or not, contributes to their skinny model bodies. Most models' personal, everyday wardrobe consists of jeans, a man-beater tank top, a pair of flats, and a leather jacket or scarf to stay warm. Let's look at how this basic outfit contributes to a supermodel body.

First, the flats. Flats help you burn calories because you walk faster and you walk more when you wear them.

Nerd Alert!

A study found that women who wear more comfortable shoes and clothing burn a minimum of 30 calories a day more than chicks strutting in stilettos or any high heels. That's 210 calories a week and 10,920 calories a year! Since it takes approximately 3,500 calories to lose a pound, we're talking about five pounds a year, just for opting out of heels! Remember that the next time you slip on some sexy heels and clothes that aren't so comfy. You want to park right by the door, don't you? You might not last as long on the dance floor, either.

When you're comfortable and your feet aren't killing you, or your clothes aren't too tight, you're a lot more likely to be active: park farther away, take the stairs, pace, dance, and so on. You're also more likely to be up for that spontaneous game of beach volleyball or that line dance everybody suddenly decides to do, or even an impromptu yoga session, because you aren't all dressed up.

However, it's also important to think about how you feel when you dress up. If you really love heels and you feel hot and sexy when you wear them, then you should wear them! What about wearing your flats to get to where you're going (the office, the party, the club), but putting on your heels right before you walk inside?

Model Behavior

People think models live in heels, but it's so not true! Part of a model's job is to see clients for casting, so in cities like New York, Milan, and Paris, we end up walking a lot. We don't have cars, so we walk to castings in flats and always change our shoes outside or down in the lobby before walking up to see the client. It's a pain in the butt in the winter in New York when there's snow everywhere. We often wear big snow boots and then stuff them into plastic bags and then into our purses. We do the same with clothes. It's freezing in New York, so we pile on the layers of warm clothes and accessories, but we have to take most of that stuff off before we see the client so we don't look ten pounds heavier than we really are (not to mention looking ridiculous all bundled up!). It's silly, really—why should we wear skimpy clothes when it's freezing outside? But the clients need to see what we look like, so that's the way it is. This is our way to compensate, because we're not going to walk through the snow in minus-five-degree weather in high heels and fashionable clothes!

Color and fit are important, too. Your clothes can actually influence how you feel about yourself. Whether you're at the gym or just modercizing, it's critical to be aware of what your clothes are doing to your body and mind. "It's important to have the right clothing to exercise in," says supermodel-actress Cheryl Tiegs. "If you throw on an old T-shirt or sweats, it's not inspiring for your workout." Models tend to wear clothes that aren't superbaggy. Fitted isn't the same as restrictive. Baggy T-shirts and sweats aren't usually very inspiring, unless you're sporting some supercute Victoria's Secret Pink getup or a hot Alternative Apparel sweat suit. But the important thing is how *you* feel in those workout clothes. If you dress like you don't like your body, that's not sexy at any size. Dress like you *love* your body, and pretty soon, you'll be rocking a yoga butt.

Color might seem like a purely aesthetic choice, but according to psychologists, it can make a difference in how your body works. Red can increase blood circulation and body temperature, which can boost workout efficiency. How? Color is just waves of light, and when these waves enter your brain through your eyes, they are converted to electrical impulses that influence your energy. Environmental psychologist David Alan Kopec, Ph.D., claims that reds and oranges raise body temperature, which can increase your energy and endurance during exercise—so put on red and orange before you hit the gym. You'll see it when you put it on, you'll catch glimpses of yourself in the mirror, and whenever you need a boost, just look down. Red, orange, wow! Instant energy! I've also seen studies that show that bright colors in general are mood boosters, so if you dress in bright colors, you might feel better, which might make you want to move even more.

And about that leather jacket and that scarf—did you know that staying warm keeps you from overeating? When it's hot outside, the last thing your body wants to do is digest a big, heavy meal. When you're cold, your body looks for ways to heat you up, and eating is a good way to do so. This also goes back to being comfortable. Models love to be comfortable, and being cold is *not* comfortable! Being too hot isn't comfortable, either, but at least heat encourages your body to drop fat, while cold encourages it to retain the fat. I've even seen a study that shows how the air conditioner can make you gain weight! It sounds crazy, but it totally makes sense. Weight-loss guru Jon Gabriel even goes so far as to suggest that you should dress and eat like you're in a tropical climate all the time to trick your body into thinking it should melt away the fat.

Other Fun Ways to Modercize

There are so many ways to modercize, and everybody has different preferences. The point of modercizing is to do what feels fun and natural to *you*. However, there are some specific ways most models like to modercize:

— **Walking.** One of the most obvious ways models modercize is by walking. We walk everywhere. Models who live in New York, Milan, Paris, and other big cities are much more likely to walk or use public transportation than to use limos or chauffeurs.

— **Shopping.** Models love to shop, but we're not hanging out in the high-priced boutiques. We love vintage! It's eco-friendly, and you get awesome designer pieces for cut-rate prices. Plus, shopping vintage means *not* maxing out your credit cards to buy clothes, which saves you from financial stress when it's time to pay the bills. Double plus: scoring the best finds means lots of calories burned digging around for the best bargains!

— **Dancing.** Models love to go dancing. It's probably our favorite pastime. Once, a bunch of us flew to Seattle for a *Vogue* show, and after the job, we all went to this pool bar across the street, and all the models were dancing like total nerds. We were laughing (stress-reducing and good for your abs!) and really letting our bodies move and be free. We didn't care what people thought of us. We just wanted to have fun. Models also love going to clubs, mostly for the dancing. That's our one splurge, where we might lose a few hours of sleep, but even when we do go out, we tend to get there, dance a lot, take some pictures, and get home long before the club closes. We even like to rock out during jobs. I have a model friend who is a DJ, and she brings the best music. We have hilarious dance sessions behind closed doors, especially when we get to wear funny outfits. Sometimes it's a mix of being delirious from being cooped up all day and just loving to dance. Either way, it's definitely modercize!

— **Making out.** Kissing is fun! And sexy! And it totally burns calories, so I think you should do it way more often!

— **Fun sports.** When models do engage in more strenuous activity, it's usually fun, not just "exercise." Popular model activities are dance classes, yoga classes, jumping rope, biking, and roller-skating. We also like activities that create more body awareness, like Pilates.

— **Cleaning.** I love to clean, and so does supermodel Marisa Miller, who says on her website that she loves doing anything domestic.

— **Playing.** Play with your kids, walk your dog, kick a ball around—whatever you love to do. Kids really help this impulse. A lot of models are moms, like übersupermodels Cindy Crawford and Kathy Ireland, as well as younger models like Jourdan Dunn, who shocked the fashion world when she got pregnant at 19 and appeared on the cover of *Teen Vogue* pregnant!

Model Behavior

You can burn tons of calories shopping, if you just shop like a model (and models are crazy about shopping—it's one of our top calorie burners!). Here are the secrets for modercizing through shopping:

- Walk like a model through those aisles! Keep your supermodel posture intact, and don't just mosey. You are on a mission to find the ultimate steal!

- Dress like a model when you shop. Forget heels. Wear flats, leggings, and comfy clothes that let you move as much as possible and shop for as long as possible.

- Use a cart. Pushing a cart burns more calories.

- Never buy something without trying it on! Seriously, you have no idea how it's going to look on your body, and trying on clothes burns an average of 150 calories an hour. Which would you rather do—try on clothes for 30 minutes or pound it out on a treadmill for 30 minutes? I vote for the clothes. (Plus, dressing-room bonuses include great lighting and good mirrors, which can boost your self-confidence.)

- Find imitations of expensive designers at places like Target. Why not save the bucks? You'll still look hot.

So here's the bottom line, Supermodel YOU—there is no one-size-fits-all way to modercize. As you cultivate self-awareness, you'll know exactly how much your body needs to move. Then all you have to do is indulge your desire for natural movement so you can get and stay in energy balance. Go ahead, move a little right now: Sit up straight, twist from side to side, roll your shoulders back. Put your headphones on and start tapping your feet or drumming on your desk. You might get in trouble with your boss or teacher, but I promise you'll feel more energized and burn a few calories while you're at it!

■ ▓ ■

CHAPTER EIGHT

Key 5: Intuitive Eating

*It's important to remember that if you don't put gas in
your car, it's going to stop. Similarly, if I don't put food
in my body, I'm going to die. I eat whatever there is to
eat because I don't want to faint on the runway*

— GISELE BÜNDCHEN, SUPERAMAZING SUPERMODEL,
SUPERMOGUL, AND SUPERMOM

If you think you need to eat like a model to get a supermodel
body, you're spot-on. But what you might not know, or might not
yet fully accept, is that models don't starve themselves. Models
eat. All the time. Fat-free? Reduced-fat? Low-carb? No way! That
stuff is fake, and it's not good for supermodel bodies. Models eat
what they want to eat, when they want to eat it—and what they
want to eat are foods that make them look and feel gorgeous,
glamorous, and *good.*

Intuitive eating means eating with self-awareness (Key 1), and
that's just what healthy models do. You don't get a supermodel
body by skipping meals, because when you don't eat, or when you
diet, your body thinks it's starving and will start to store everything you eat as fat, even if it's just a salad. This was how our ancestors survived food shortages and famines, but that's obviously
not a problem in most industrialized nations anymore. But you
already know that.

And you know that now, we have plenty of food to go around, and around it goes—around our thighs, around our butts, and around our tummies. Whenever you skip a meal or wait too long to eat, you activate that fat-storage mode, so instead of using that muffin you had for breakfast as energy, your body turns it into a muffin top.

The way this works is totally ironic. The more you starve yourself, the more your body thinks you're starving; and the more fat you gain, the less you eat. So unfair! But the upside is that eating more often will actually help you *lose weight*. It's a huge mistake dieters make, and the reason why models don't diet. Dieting makes you fat! No model wants to be stuck in fat-storage mode! No model can afford to have a muffin top.

So we eat often, and we eat according to what our bodies need. We listen to our bodies, and we give them what they want. When you are self-aware, you eat according to your needs because you're more in touch with yourself and able to distinguish the difference between the environmental cues that make you eat (like being tired, bored, upset, or working in a cubicle next to the girl who keeps a bowl of candy on her desk) and internal cues that tell you when you're truly hungry.

For example, the smell of food can trigger emotions and stimulate hormones that make you want to eat. Companies use the power of aromatherapy to lure you in and "brand" you. Ever walked past an Abercrombie store? They pump Abercrombie cologne all over that store; just walking past one will intoxicate you. Oscar de la Renta sprayed every model with their new perfume before we went down the runway. It's no different with food companies. They want you to eat more because that means they make more cash. Why else do you think they put out all those food samples in the grocery store on the weekends? Have you ever driven by a restaurant, smelled the food cooking, and just had to stop, even though you had no thoughts of food before you smelled that smell? These places should have signs that say SMELLER BEWARE, not BUYER BEWARE! (Or both!)

The fashion designer Karl Lagerfeld once said something about how if he smelled food, he wouldn't need to eat it. Sometimes I do this—I purposely inhale and enjoy the aroma of food, and let that be enough, if I know I'm not really hungry. You can do this, too—whenever you pass a bakery or a barbecue place or a doughnut shop, check in with your own hunger and tap into your self-awareness. Are you really hungry, or is it just the smell? Can you just enjoy the pleasure of that incredible smell without all the problems that come from actually eating the doughnut?

I will often walk into Starbucks and smell the coffee and want one. And sometimes, I do have coffee. But most of the time, coffee is not good for me. It makes me jittery. It almost always upsets my stomach. It picks me up and makes me hyper for like an hour, and then it drops me faster than a roller coaster at Magic Mountain. It makes me pee incessantly. It makes my breath stink and stains my pearly-white teeth. So most of the time, just smelling that amazing coffee smell is good enough for me.

I'm not saying that I don't succumb to coffee now and then, because sometimes I do. And when I do, I own it, I love it, and I enjoy it. But 80 percent or more of the time, I will just smell it, and let my mind and body relive the coffee experience. My body will remember the negatives, and then I know I don't want to go there, so when the barista asks me what I'd like, I'm most likely to say, "A venti hot tea, please. Thank you!"

Try this! Do you like coffee? Do you even like the taste of coffee, or is it really the taste of the cream and/or sugar or other sweeteners (aka calories) you load in there? How will you feel if you drink it? This is all part of self-awareness.

Sometimes, I just enjoy the smell of food I have no intention of eating. Like steak. I love the smell of steak cooking, but I would never eat it because I'm a vegan and I haven't had steak since I was probably ten years old. But guess what I do love? My dad! And guess who used to make steak and potatoes all the time?

I associate the smell of steak with love and with my dad, and it makes me happy, not actually hungry, like I might first think if I weren't self-aware. It's the same with the smell of barbecue. I love this smell! But what does a raw vegan eat on a barbecue? Nothing, that's what! Still, the smell of barbecue reminds me of summer, family, friends, and good times, and all of that makes me happy, too.

The sight of food can be just as enticing as the smell, and studies have proved that you eat more if you're exposed to the sight of delicious food. So put it out of sight—out of sight, out of mind. For instance, don't stand by the food at parties, and don't walk by the bakery (sight and smell—a double whammy!). Sometimes you can't avoid food in your face and scents in your nose, and that's when you need to check in with the Five Keys and your hunger, and decide if it's something you really want. Doughnuts, cupcakes, candy, pastries, cakes, and all those things always look appealing and smell delicious to me, and sometimes I might indulge, but I pretty much know that I'm just eating sugar and not much else. Sugar has been shown to age the body, and everybody knows models have to stay forever young! Plus, sugar will throw your blood sugar out of whack. I know that when I eat really sugary food I'm like a kid on crack. Sometimes I might go for it anyway, but more often than not, I'll pass, and if I'm still hungry, I'll go for fruit or stevia-sweetened iced tea first. That's usually enough to put the sugar monster back in the closet.

So even if you see or smell unhealthy food, recognize that it's going to try to entice you, but be wise. Know how it will make you feel afterward. Let the sight and smell intoxicate you, but not beyond reason. Keep in mind what's really going on inside you. Is it hunger? Or is it something else? And whether or not you eat or drink it doesn't matter, as long as you know why, and as long as you decide with conscious awareness.

Eating with self-awareness is the key to intuitive eating. You aren't following a meal plan, because you don't *need* to follow a meal plan. You know your own body and your own hunger signals well enough to tell the difference between fake hunger and real hunger. And when you're really hungry, you eat.

Being self-aware and eating intuitively also means that sometimes, a little bit of something that's supposedly "bad" can be just fine, and if you really want it, you should enjoy it! I'll never forget standing outside the office of the "new faces" director at my agency in Paris, overhearing one of the models I was living with in the model apartment bawling her eyes out. She was having trouble with her weight (or so this agent believed), and I knew she hardly ate anything. Apparently, the agent had seen her eating chocolate, and was yelling at her. She said, and I quote, "Models don't eat chocolate!"

That poor girl. This is a totally untrue statement! A lot of models eat chocolate. They even eat McDonald's! (Supermodel Gisele Bündchen was actually discovered at a McDonald's in Brazil when she was 13.) But they don't binge or eat monster meals. Instead, models use some special tricks to keep themselves satisfied without packing in more calories than they need (so they stay in energy balance).

They also do some really expected things. Obvious things. Things you already know. Things you probably don't do. Let's start with those.

SUPERMODEL **SAYS . . .**

Last year I was kind of stressed, so this year I came prepared. I brought my own peanut butter and jelly sandwich because it's something that really calms me down. I also have homeopathic stress reliever drops that I've used a few times as well as some yoga breathing.

— Lindsay Ellingson, supermodel and real-life angel, in regard to prepping for the annual Victoria's Secret runway show (as quoted in Modelinia, a popular fashion blog)

So Tell Me Something I Don't Know

Every freaking diet book, doctor, nutritionist, and expert has the same advice. I'm not talking about the crazy gimmicks like leaving out major food groups or doing something strange. I'm just talking about basic, commonsense pieces of advice. I call them the No-Brainer Diet Rules. But even though I doubt we've missed something the last hundred times we've heard these, let's review.

The No-Brainer Diet Rules

The rules everybody knows and that people still don't follow—except models!

— **Eat breakfast.** How many times have you heard this? If you're still not eating breakfast after everything you've read and everything you know, then you must not really want to be skinny! The only time I advocate skipping breakfast is if you're fasting, which can be a healthy thing to do once in a while, as long as you do it the right way.

— **Snack.** OMG, how many times can someone mention the importance of snacking? Eat an apple, a handful of almonds, a bag of carrots, blah, blah, blah. Have them with you all the time, just in case you get hungry. The three model must-haves are water, snacks, and a cell phone, so bring snacks for when you don't have any other healthy choices. Duh.

SUPERMODEL **SAYS . . .**

You have to eat regularly to maintain your energy levels. If you starve your body, it simply stores everything that you do eat.

— Cindy Crawford, übersupermodel, supermogul, and supermom (as quoted on **www.beautyden.com**)

— **Drink water.** Yeah, yeah, we know! Drink half your body weight in ounces, or drink two cups before every meal, or whatever. The point is that we should all be drinking more, and there are plenty of ways to make water more appealing, like drinking flavored water. You've probably also heard that people mistake thirst for hunger, so try drinking water before you stuff your face with something you don't really want. Water is crucial for losing weight, but it's also crucial for beauty. A dehydrated face isn't pretty.

SUPERMODEL **SAYS . . .**

I drink approximately 64 ounces of water a day to stay hydrated, and I also love coconut water. When I need a little energy pick-me-up, I reach for tea (my fave is green tea), and I have Sleepytime Tea (chamomile) to help me relax at the end of the day. By the way, cold green tea bags are great for bags under your eyes.

— Melissa Rose Haro, *Sports Illustrated* Rookie of the Year swimsuit model, 2008–2009

— **Avoid empty calories**. What are empty calories, anyway? They are calories with little to no nutritional value. Most of us continue to stuff in the empty calories, like soda, mocha lattes, white bread, and sugar. It might be fun in the moment, but the price of empty calories is a body loaded down with fat you don't need or want, and devoid of the nutrients you do need. Models eat and drink with purpose. We know that healthy food gives us sustained energy, water makes us pretty, and nutrient-dense foods like berries and fresh veggies contain antioxidants that make us look and feel better.

— **Don't eat late at night**. This topic is a little controversial, but seriously, if you think about it for yourself, it's pretty obvious. Food is energy. Do you need energy to go to bed? Hello? How basic is that? Forget all the other reasons why eating late is bad—the bottom line is that most people confuse being tired with being hungry. Just go to bed already! If you absolutely have to eat, stick to protein and fat, never carbs like popcorn or cookies. If you don't give your body carbs at night, it will burn fat while you sleep. If you give it a little bit of fat, that encourages the fat-burning process.

Model Pretty

Fat does not make you fat! Fat makes you beautiful. Fat is essential for maintaining a thin physique and a pretty face, but you need to eat the right fats, like the ones in nuts, seeds, avocados, and fish, rather than the ones from fatty meats and dairy products.

Because I'm a vegan, and fruits and vegetables aren't exactly dripping with fat, I'm obsessed with consuming fat. I actually drink oil! Pumpkin oil is one of my favorites, and I also eat spoonfuls of coconut oil, or use it like butter. And it's not just me! Supermodel Miranda Kerr, for example, says she puts coconut oil in her green tea for breakfast, and that coconut oil is her secret to clear skin, shiny hair, and a trim figure. She eats four tablespoons a day.

The first time I ever did a showroom was for Céline in New York. I was the oldest girl there, but everyone thought I was the youngest, even though a lot of the models were teenagers. I've seen 16-year-old models who look 10 years older than they are and already have wrinkles because they never eat fat. I also did a *Teen Vogue* fashion show that year and fit right in with the girls, some of whom were 13! I owe it all to keeping plenty of healthy fat in my diet.

— **Sleep**. Speaking of going to bed, not sleeping enough is probably the biggest reason people gain weight. We covered this when we talked about Key 2, but just as a reminder: When you don't get enough sleep, you really jack up your body in more ways than one. Lack of sleep will eventually lead to weight gain; plus, it makes you uglier and grumpier. Let's see, rolls on your thighs and bags under your eyes, or a fresh face and a tight bod? Hmm, such a tough decision. . . .

— **Eat slower**. The research is there in black and white: eat slower and you'll automatically consume fewer calories. Slow eaters consume up to 70 fewer calories. Multiply that by all your meals and you're looking at around 20 pounds a year of weight loss, just from slowing down! How many times have you heard this? We should be slow chewers, not slow learners!

> ## MODEL **TALK**
>
> *Chewing prevents bloating. Chew food until it is like apple-sauce in your mouth. Digestion begins in the mouth, and better-digested food means less gas and bloating.*
>
> — Dr. Joseph Mercola, super–alternative physician

— **Don't diet**. It's not that diets don't work, because most *will* make you lose weight. The problem with diets is that they're a quick fix, and once you return to your normal life, you almost always gain the weight back and then some. Not to mention that diets totally screw up your metabolism. How many books these days say "Stop dieting forever" or some riff on that theme? About a million.

— **Choose real food.** A lot of models are total health nuts. We love whole, organic food; we snack on fruit, nuts, and protein bars; and we love salads, soup, fresh juice and smoothies, raw food, and homemade dishes. If you ditch the processed crap and focus on the food the earth provides for us (as free from chemicals as possible)—and you focus on self-awareness when you eat, so you learn to feel what and how much your body wants—then you're going to be in a good place, nutritionally. You won't ever have to think about a diet.

So you already knew all of those rules. Why did I bother repeating them? Two reasons:

1. You aren't following them.
2. Models *are* following them.

So what's the problem? You say you want a supermodel body, but you don't follow these obvious, basic rules? Are you some kind of diet criminal that you have to break the rules? Maybe you should be arrested!

Do you wear white after Labor Day? Women are more likely to follow fashion rules than these No-Brainer Diet Rules—but why? Would you rather be fashionable than have the body of your dreams? Why are people more likely to go on some crazy diet than adhere to these simple recommendations that require little to no effort?

I can't tell you how many times I've been on the other end of someone going off about how they want to lose weight and don't know what to do, and my first question is always "Do you eat breakfast?" I'm amazed every time, because the answer is very often no! No? Are you sure you *really* want to lose weight? This is not rocket science . . . it's common sense!

Worst of all, the people who complain that they can't lose weight know these rules. They can recite them faster than a model can say her ABCs, but they still don't follow them. Even if they do happen to eat breakfast or abide by a few of the rules, they are almost always in some kind of No-Brainer Diet Rule violation.

Most of the models and skinny girls in general whom I know follow these rules. They might have a hard time following the law—Naomi Campbell, Kate Moss, and Paris Hilton, for example, have all had their run-ins with the legal system—but for the most part, they don't break the No-Brainer Diet Rules. Why not? Because maintaining a certain body size is a necessity for them. A model's job requires her to be a certain size. Being tall, skinny, and pretty doesn't mean that you'll necessarily get the job, but not fitting into the clothes is a definite deal breaker.

With Paris Hilton and the other skinny celebs, if they were overweight or chubby, would we still obsess about them as much? Poor celebrities can't gain a pound, even when they're pregnant, without the paparazzi slamming them for it. So channel that inner supermodel. Pretend your career depends on staying thin and healthy. Pretend the paparazzi are stalking you and recording every extra pound and fat roll for the world to see—front-page news! Because even if your career doesn't depend on this, your health does! If you want to be skinny, you've got to follow the No-Brainer Diet Rules. Period.

There are reasons why these rules work. Each rule comes with its own set of good reasons, but by far the most important one is that if you religiously follow the No-Brainer Diet Rules, your body will find its balance. You'll be able to splurge on pizza or ice cream now and then, and you'll be fine because your body will be able to handle it. It won't be busy recovering from diet abuse, starvation, bingeing, or whatever else you might have been doing to it before. You'll be in energy balance. You'll regain your self-awareness (Key 1).

SUPERMODEL **SAYS . . .**

I never count calories. I know that what I'm putting into my body is good for me, and that's all that really matters. I eat slowly, and I never overeat. Leftovers rock—why eat it all at once and feel sick to your stomach? Soda is a never. Did you know the average teenager in America eats something like 48 teaspoons of sugar a day? Gross. Why not enjoy a nice glass of iced tea with a little lemon and maybe sweetened with some honey, or even better, some water with some fresh berries or lemon and cucumber? (You'll feel like you're at a spa!)

— Dani Lundquist, international fashion model

Your Supermodel Motivation

I think the real reason why models tend to follow the No-Brainer Diet Rules while other people don't is that having a good body is more important to models—that's the bottom line. But you can make your body and health a priority if you just decide to do it. You have to realize how important it is that you have the body you want. It's superficial in a sense to say that having the body of your dreams will make you happier, but in some ways it's true, because having a healthy body means you'll have more energy and you'll feel better, and that reflects on everything in your life.

Plus, think of all the negativity you can ditch! Think about how much time you spend obsessing over your weight. Think about how unhappy you are because you can't seem to lose those extra pounds or because you can't fit into your favorite jeans anymore. It's not about being skinny or fat; it's about being confident and happy in the body you have. There are plenty of curvier women out there who swear they're happy, and if they are, and they're healthy too, that's all that matters. That's all this is about.

The skinny girls everyone envies are not just thin, they're happy. They're confident. Most important, they're healthy and vibrant. Obviously, we've seen the media exploit certain celebrities and models who have had and still may have eating disorders, but we don't want to look like them—we want to be thin and fit, not walking skeletons.

Just consider how not having the body of your dreams is affecting you, then decide that for you, it *is* a matter of your job, your health, the reflection in the mirror, and your *life*. You have to have the body you want—and you should be able to have it!

Model Behavior

People constantly blame the media, and especially models, for setting this so-called unrealistic standard that every girl seems to want, but that's just absurd! I attempted my toothbrush-gagging way before I ever saw my first copy of *Vogue* magazine. Research proves that young girls get their body-image issues primarily from their mothers, not from the media. No surprise to me, considering my mom and I were *Sweating to the Oldies* with Richard Simmons when I was two years old! I loved doing his videos with my mom. I was just a little girl, so for me, it was a blast. Little did I know that this was just the beginning of a lifelong obsession with my body.

And I might have learned some dysfunctional body-image stuff from my mom, but thankfully, I turned it into a positive passion. For many women, however, it turns negative and chips away at their self-esteem and confidence, year after year. I think most women have some level of body obsession. Who doesn't want to have a great body, be healthy, and feel good in their own skin? There's nothing wrong with that. You just have to *want it enough.*

Beyond the No-Brainer Diet Rules

So now you know why models follow the obvious rules—but now, let's get to some secrets. There are some things models do, in addition to following the No-Brainer Diet Rules, to keep their eating under control. I call them the 11 Secrets to a Supermodel Body.

11 Secrets to a Supermodel Body

1. Eat pretty. One of the most effective strategies that models employ is to eat pretty. That means they choose smaller portions, use smaller plates, take smaller bites, chew their food slowly and thoroughly (with mouths closed!), and are generally aware of how they look when they eat.

In fact, we're so aware of it that it can get really annoying when we're backstage at a show getting our hair done or something else, and we're simultaneously trying to get a bite to eat and some photographer has a camera in our faces! It's like these people want to document the "rare" sight of a model eating, when actually, we eat constantly—when we have the chance. I've seen so many models yell at photographers for this. It's funny, but it's also rude! It's like, "Dude, can you let me eat in peace? As if it's not crazy enough that I've got rollers in my hair and someone painting my toenails! Back off!"

For weight loss, however, knowing how you look when you eat and trying to eat pretty is really effective. If you're shoveling it in, you're not going to look pretty, but if you think about looking pretty when you eat, you're going to eat less, and you'll give your brain a chance to keep up with your stomach. It takes about 20 minutes for your brain to realize you're full, so the slower you eat, the better chance you have to notice this instead of barreling right on past the "I'm full now" cues your body is sending you. Eating pretty is like a direct line to self-awareness!

Model Behavior

One great way to apply Key 1 (self-awareness) to Key 5 (intuitive eating) is to learn how to distinguish between psychological hunger and physical hunger. Physical hunger is real hunger, when your stomach growls and even the healthiest food sounds delicious because you really haven't eaten for a while. Psychological hunger is much different, is more unpredictable, and comes on suddenly, often driven by some sort of emotion. Identifying these emotions is the key you need in order to get a lockdown on psychological hunger, and self-awareness is the only way to do it.

Start by noticing your most intense hungers and cravings, including what you crave and in what kind of situation. For example, I get the desire to eat when I'm stressed. I made this connection by asking myself why. WTH? I'll be running late—i.e., stressing—and find myself in the fridge or cupboard, which is crazy! First, I'm late, I need to go, so why do I think I suddenly have time to indulge in a leisurely snack? Second, I know myself well enough to know that I definitely do not want to stuff something in my mouth and walk out the door. It's so funny to me every time it happens and I catch myself.

Once I developed this awareness, it helped me a lot to avoid this. Not always—sometimes I still do it—but it gave me the awareness to recognize it and stop it before it goes too far.

So when you get superhungry, question that hunger. Is it real? Is it really about food? Or is it about something else? (If you're really into this, check out Doreen Virtue's awesome book I mentioned in Chapter 4, *Constant Craving,* where you can look up the psychological reasons behind all your specific food cravings.)

2. Buddy up. Models may have a hard time with long-term relationships because of the nature of our work, but we've all taken a sort of unspoken vow to support each other when it comes to food. We remind each other not to eat late at night, to pay attention to food labels, and to make good choices that will keep our energy up. We also like to share entrées when dining out because restaurants serve portion sizes that are way too huge.

This is significant: studies show that when your friends are overweight, you're more likely to be overweight. The opposite is also true: when models hang out together, they're more likely to help keep each other in good shape, just because of peer pressure!

I'm not saying ditch all your friends who struggle with weight, because you can be a good example for *them,* but I am saying it's a good idea to also get some friends who are committed to healthy eating rather than dysfunctional eating. When you're around them, you'll be more likely to want to eat like they do, and that's great for your supermodel body. Be with people who encourage you.

MODEL **TALK**

You must constantly ask yourself these questions: Who am I around? What are they doing to me? What have they got me reading? What have they got me saying? Where do they have me going? What do they have me thinking? And most important, what do they have me becoming? Then ask yourself the big question: Is that okay? Your life does not get better by chance, it gets better by change.

— Jim Rohn, super–motivational speaker and author

3. Follow the Rule of Fist. I've always heard that it's a "rule of thumb" not to eat more food in one sitting than the size of your fist. So why call it a rule of thumb? I call it the Rule of Fist! Your stomach really isn't all that big, so if you never eat more than a fist-size portion of food at any meal, you won't overstuff yourself and you'll naturally limit your intake without counting calories. Small plates can help you feel like you're eating more.

Model Behavior

I once read this fascinating article about how sumo wrestlers eat. You know, those giant Japanese wrestlers who smack each other with their enormous bellies? Sumo wrestlers only eat twice a day. They skip breakfast, they train all morning on no food, then they eat a giant lunch. By the time they get food, their bodies are in major fat-storage mode, so everything they eat adds to their bulk. They eat a lot of meat, rice, and vegetables, and drink beer. Then, they eat their last giant meal right before they go to bed, so all that food gets stored as fat when they sleep.

> It's a great recipe if you want to be huge and fat—and it's almost exactly the opposite of what models do. If you want to have a supermodel body, you have to eat breakfast, eat before you exercise, eat a lot of small meals and snacks instead of a few giant ones, and not eat right before you go to bed.

4. Downsize. When ordering, always get the small. The small latte, the small soda, the small fries, the small muffin. Make it your "thing." Large is just so . . . *large.* You can always go back for more, but you might find, especially if you are eating with self-awareness, that the small size was enough, even though you would have plowed through a large latte, soda, fries, or muffin without even realizing it was too much. Go small, especially if you're going for a smaller booty or a smaller tummy, and savor every bite so you slow down.

To take it one step further, most of the cool new, trendy fast-food places are also health centered or at least healthier, like Chipotle and FroYo. Honestly, with a model mind-set, you can even eat at Mickey D's and choose the healthier options, like salads, fruit, and oatmeal for breakfast (but ask for the no-sugar version—the standard is loaded with sugar). Just don't overindulge, order the small (or even the "kids' meal," which has plenty of calories for the average adult), chew thoroughly, eat pretty, and *never* supersize!

5. Snack like a supermodel. Ask any model to open up her purse and you will find a trove of . . . makeup? Nope. Food. We stash snacks everywhere. Seriously—no model wants to get caught without food. The biggest reason is that we listen to our bodies, and we know when we need to eat. When we have our own food, we can control when we eat and what we eat, instead of having to rely on other people catering our jobs and events. Sometimes the catered food on a job is great and healthy and exactly what we want, and sometimes it's terrible or doesn't come when we're hungry . . . or doesn't come at all. Models always run across the stereotype that we don't eat, so we don't always get fed! Or we're just too busy traveling or working to stop and eat. During times like these, healthy snacks are all we're going to get. And the snacks have to be healthy, because unhealthy snacks just aren't satisfying for as long as we need them to be to hold us over until the next meal.

Model Behavior

Some of the most common snacks that models eat:

- Kale chips
- Nuts
- Protein bars
- Fresh juices
- Protein shakes
- Fruit
- Yogurt

---

6. Eat chic. Today, it's all about food that is eco-friendly, organic, natural, and fresh. It happens to be *très chic* to eat this way, and models are *always* up on what's cool. That's why models love to pick up food at farmers' markets. In fact, buying and eating "local" or "green" is a favorite model pastime. If you're eating green, you're probably eating healthful and natural foods grown purely and with love. That's better for your supermodel body, and you're totally on trend!

When was the last time you saw an article in *Vogue* about how chic and posh it was to eat at McDonald's or how the latest rage is eating Snickers bars and Doritos (even though they recently put Snickers bars "on a diet" and are making them smaller!)? Too much of that stuff isn't healthy, and unhealthy is not chic. Models shop at Whole Foods and Trader Joe's because places like these are current and in! It's where you'll find food that's healthier than the food at your average supermarket (although with a supermodel mind-set, you can shop for food anywhere and still make healthy choices).

Another reason models like to shop at farmers' markets is because walking through the market, enjoying the great outdoors, and lifting bags of produce are great ways to modercize (Key 4)!

7. Choose beauty foods. Some foods have special beauty-enhancing properties, and models know this and choose these foods more often. These foods, especially plant foods, contain beautifying antioxidants and hundreds of thousands of phytochemicals that increase health and beauty. Scientists have only identified a tiny percentage of them, but we know they are there. Let them work for you! Put color back in your cheeks and get shiny hair, bright eyes, and clearer skin by choosing these beauty foods whenever you can.

Model Behavior

Top Ten Supermodel Beauty Foods:

1. Berries (blueberries, strawberries, raspberries, blackberries, acai berries, etc.)

2. Leafy greens (spinach, kale, Swiss chard, etc.)

3. Nuts (walnuts, almonds, cashews, etc.)

4. Citrus fruit (oranges, grapefruits, mandarins, lemons, limes, etc.)

5. Good fats (olive oil, coconut oil, avocados, flaxseed oil)

6. Herbs/spices (especially oregano, turmeric, cayenne, cinnamon, and ginger)

7. Chocolate (preferably dark or raw)

8. Fish/seafood (especially salmon) and sea vegetables (like seaweed)

9. Tomatoes

10. Water!

---

8. No fakes, no freebies. In general, models never count calories, and avoid not-natural foods, like margarine, Twinkies, or white bread, unless we *really* want them. And then, we just have a few bites. We avoid empty calories, and we steer way clear of anything fake or "free"!

If it's fat-free, calorie-free, carb-free, or imitation-whatever, we're not interested. Here are some other free-food traps:

- Free doughnuts at work. (Do you really want them?)

- Free Starbucks run. (Do you really want/need that mocha latte?)

- Free M&Ms at the doctor's office. (Who's been touching them, and what kind of germs do they have?)

- Free samples at the grocery store. (Just decide they're gross and leave them alone!)

SUPERMODEL **SAYS . . .**

My main thing is not eating processed food.

— Marisa Miller, supergorgeous supermodel and surfer girl
(via **www.fittipdaily.com**)

9. Follow the Rule of 20. Models remember the Rule of 20, which comes in three parts:

- *The 80/20 Rule:* 80 percent of your weight is based on what you eat, and only 20 percent is based on how much you exercise.

- *The 20-Minute Rule:* It takes 20 minutes for your body to register that you have eaten, so you have to eat slowly and pay attention. Give your body time to realize when you are actually full.

- *The 20-Day Rule:* It takes your body about 20 days to develop a routine or habit, so if you're changing something about your life, like your eating habits or movement habits, you need to give it at least 20 days to really set in!

Model Behavior

People gain an average of five pounds during the holiday season, but that doesn't have to be you. Self-awareness will help you eat intuitively, so you'll only eat what you want and as much as you need in order to stay in energy balance. If you do end up eating more, your body will feel like moving more, and your weight will stay right where it belongs.

10. Live in a no-crash zone. "Help, I need a ride into town! Preferably in a car that will crash, because I don't really care if I get there or not. . . ."

This is how I see crash dieting. The name says it all! A crash diet, like a car crash, is not going to get you where you need or want to be. But it will come with *a lot* of side effects. Think about what happens when you get into a car crash: possible injuries, or even death; a smashed-up car; the insurance hike; the time delay to get where you were going; and so on. People think that if they drive superfast or recklessly, they might save time, but it often takes *more* time, and you risk an accident and a speeding ticket, too. Losing weight is the same way.

I also think of crash dieting as a little like hitting a runway before getting to see it. You're totally unprepared, and that can be bad for your performance. Just the other day at an Oscar de la Renta show, one of the models was missing while we were doing the show run-through. That's where we rehearse the show—the lineup, the pace, and so forth—on the runway before the audience gets there, and usually before hair and makeup. We all knew she was going to be in trouble during the show.

It's rare that you don't get to see the runway first, although this happens and it can be scary! Sometimes I have no idea what the runway looks like or feels like. Not all runways are straight. Some have stairs. Some go in circles. Some are crazy slippery, and so on. I never saw or walked the runway before my Dolce & Gabbana show in Milan, and I was terrified when I stepped out. It was all mirrors and bright lights. I couldn't see anything because I was blinded by light. Literally! This is pretty common, especially at the end of the runway where you stop and pose. It's usually so freaking bright, and all these cameras are flashing and you can barely open your eyes, let alone see the runway or where you're supposed to stop. This makes for a lot of laughs when models walk off the end of the runway. Yep! This happens a lot, actually! Fortunately, most of the time they don't get hurt too badly.

This is like life. You never know what's going to happen, so you have to be ready with good nutrition and self-awareness, not starvation and crash diets that will *make* you crash, at least metaphorically. If you're starving yourself or crash dieting all the time, you're not going to be in shape to handle life's little surprises. Models have to be energized and bikini-ready all the time. We can't afford quick fixes that compromise us. So forget the quick fixes, and fix your habits for good instead. It might take longer to get there, but at least you'll know you're really going to get there—hopefully without falling off the end of a runway!

Model Behavior

A lot of models do occasional short fasts or cleanses, and a lot of non-models do them, too. Fasting and cleansing can be great ways to clear your system of toxic buildup, like bad bacteria that thrive on too much sugar. However, cleanses and fasts should never be used for weight loss. They are simply for resetting your system. Make sure that any fast longer than one or two days is undertaken with the supervision of a medical professional, and that you drink tons of water and fresh juice during your fast so you don't damage your body.

---

11. Write it down. Who has time to keep long-winded journals about food? Not models, but what a lot of us do is just write down what we eat, or record it on our computers or phones through a cool app. Although a lot of my model friends say they never count calories, I do. As I've mentioned, I keep careful track of what I eat, mostly to make sure I eat enough and get enough protein. But it also helps hone my self-awareness, so I recommend this for everyone.

Write down every bite you eat, and also how you felt about it before and after. The best way to do this is to use an app that will tell you the calorie count and the nutritional value of your foods. A lot of them also let you log your exercise (or modercize, as the case may be), so you can see how your calorie burn stacks up against your calorie intake. This is crucial for staying in energy balance and for cultivating your food knowledge, as well as your self-awareness. A lot of studies have demonstrated that when people write down what they eat, they tend to eat less and make better, more nutritious food choices.

It's so easy to eat mindlessly, but if you keep track of it all, you've engaged your awareness, and then you're more likely to realize that you don't necessarily want to eat as much as you were going to eat. It's also about becoming aware of the effects that food has on you. You might not realize that sugar makes you cranky or caffeine makes you jumpy or fruit makes you feel really clean and energized unless you start writing it down. I talked about all of this in Chapter 4, so you might want to look back there for a refresher, but the point is that you have to give your body what it needs to thrive, not what makes it tired and sluggish. To do that, you have to notice which foods make you feel like a supermodel, and which make you feel like a slug. Then, you'll have the power to choose accordingly.

So just write it down, and you'll start training yourself to pay attention. It's not about guilt. It's not even about forcing you to measure your food or count calories or any of that. It's just about self-awareness. (Check out Appendix B for some free apps you can install on your phone to help you.)

■ ■

The bottom line is just this: models eat, and you should, too, with self-awareness, restraint, and total enjoyment. Start right now—why waste one more second being anything less than Supermodel YOU? Just follow the No-Brainer Diet Rules and the 11 Secrets to a Supermodel Body, and your body is going to start doing exactly what you want it to do, feeling like you want it to feel, and looking like you've always dreamed it could look. Food is the way, so kick your intuition into gear and watch your body transform.

■ ■ ■

CHAPTER NINE

Modelize Your Life

*The more you see yourself as what you'd like to become,
and act as if what you want is already there, the more
you'll activate those dormant forces that will collaborate
to transform your dream into your reality.*

— DR. WAYNE W. DYER, SUPERAMAZING SELF-HELP GURU

Every model dreams about getting her wings. Her Victoria's Secret wings, that is. Earning your VS wings is a huge honor—that, and getting into the *Sports Illustrated* swimsuit issue are the most coveted jobs in modeling. So those wings are hard to come by, and very few girls ever get them.

But you can have your own wings—the metaphorical wings that will allow you to reach your dreams! All you have to know is how to "modelize" your life.

Okay, I know you might be suspicious of that word, especially if you know that a *modelizer* is the term for a man (or a woman, I suppose) who only sleeps with models. That is *so* not what I'm talking about here! In my world, modelizing your life means using the Five Keys to transform it to "super" status. I want you to start feeling like your very own version of a supermodel, and this is the way.

In the last few chapters, I talked about each of the Five Keys, and I told you how models use them, how I use them, and a little bit about how you can use them. In this chapter, we're going to focus on *you*—what you need to know, where your head is, and where you want to go. I'm going to ask you lots of questions, and I want you to give serious thought to the answers, because this is where *Supermodel YOU* gets personal. Along the way, I'll give you more tips, tricks, and strategies you can use to modelize your life. You're going to start feeling different—and looking different, too. You're going to get into energy balance, and your body, mind, and life are going to start getting primed. It's exciting! And fun! And it all begins with knowing exactly where you want to go.

I'm not dumb. I know that you are probably reading this book because you want to lose weight. You're like, "Okay, Sarah De-Anna, tell me how to be more self-aware and sleep more and blah, blah, blah, but just be sure it's going to help me get a supermodel body."

Okay! I hear you! Every single one of the Five Keys will get you there, even if it seems like an indirect road to a fabulous bod. It's more direct than you think.

But first, you're going to have to own that slammin' body of yours, awesome parts and not-so-awesome parts included. We all have insecurities and negative thoughts about our bodies. Forget what size dress you wear. Who cares? If it fits well, that means you look awesome! Forget the number on the scale. When you practice the Five Keys, it's going to slide down to where you want it eventually, but obsessing about it will just distract you from living your best life possible right now. When I step on the scale, I tell the *scale* what number I want to see, and whatever it tells me back is just a message about whether I'm in balance or not. Isn't that the original purpose of a scale—for balance?

Owning your body and loving it is also about accepting the now of your body. Moles, frizzy hair, big nose, gangly limbs, flat butt, huge feet, bony elbows, chubby knees . . . all of it and any of it that has to do with *you*. People used to say that supermodel Gisele Bündchen had a big nose, that Tyra Banks had a forehead that was too large, that Cindy Crawford's mole was a problem, and, of course, that the legendary Lauren Hutton should fix that famous gap between her teeth. Now just look at all of them! If Gisele or any of the others had let someone else's criticism about them affect their decision to go for a modeling career, they might never have become the legends they are today. Those women owned who they were and embraced their beauty, and now everyone else embraces them, too.

One of the best pieces of advice I ever got was from top model Michelle Buswell. I had just started working, and she was already a star. She told me how she used to have really bad acne, and our current agency didn't even want to represent her. But she stuck it out. She didn't give up. She made them love her as much as she loved herself. She told me you *have* to love yourself—everything about yourself! "My armpit fat," she said as she pinched her under-arm. "I love it!" This is exactly why she's so beautiful.

It doesn't mean you can't change things. It just means you know who you are and where you are, how you feel, and how much it matters to you to move in a different direction. And then to love it all—the imperfections, and the process of change, too. You are a supercool work in progress, so don't miss a minute of getting to hang out with, understand, and love yourself.

Here's the bottom line: if you think you look like crap, then you're going to feel like crap, and then everybody is going to per-ceive you that way. Do you really want to be a crappy person? But if you feel like a million dollars—if you feel like a supermodel walking into a room—then heads will turn, no matter what your dress size is, no matter where you have a mole. Even if you have armpit fat. Let your self-awareness feed your self-love, and you'll be halfway there.

But first, you're going to have to stop hiding from the truth. If you don't know where you are and what you've got, you don't know what you have to work with. So let's get some things down on paper and in the forefront of your mind before I start telling you what you can do to make it happen. Remember: self-awareness! It's everything! If you want to change your body and your life, you have to be totally self-aware about where you are *right now*. Got it?

Mapping Your Dream Body

Now, this is going to take some prep work, because before you can plan your journey, you have to know where you are and what your destination really is. And it has to be *your* destination, not mine or some other model's or a movie star's or whoever's. *Yours.* So, the first job is to figure out what a supermodel body means for you. Because of course *your* supermodel body will be unique, just like the rest of you! This is the most important part of getting and keeping the body of your dreams.

It's time to sit down, calm down, and think for a minute. I want you to picture your dream body. I want you to think about the number on the scale you would like to see (or better yet, about a five-pound range where you'd like to hang out). Then I want you to think about the shape you'd like to have. Would you like to trim a bit off the backside? Tighten up your upper arms? Flatten the belly? Close your eyes and try to picture how you would like your body to look. Don't focus so much on all the stuff you don't like or don't want. Focus on the image of the body you *do* want, one that makes you feel good and strong and sexy and beautiful. Maybe you'll fill in the picture with some other aspects, too, like a different hairstyle or nice skin or whatever. It's your picture; it's your vision, so you can make it into anything *you* really want to be. It's super YOU!

Now, let me warn you that some stuff is probably going to get in your way when you try to do this. You might be distracted by thinking about other people's bodies, and while that's okay for inspiration, remember that you're thinking about *your* body here. You need to be a little bit realistic—if you're 5′4″, all the self-awareness in the world won't make you 5′10″. If you have broad shoulders or narrow hips or big feet, they are what they are. But that doesn't mean you can't totally optimize and rock out the body you've got! Any height, any shape, any quality can be totally knockout gorgeous when it's optimized.

The other things you have to watch out for are the stories you tell yourself. We all have these. They are the ideas we believe about our lives and our bodies, like *I inherited my mother's thunder thighs* or *I'm Italian, so I'll always be bigger* or *I've always been a chubby girl, and I always will be.* These are just stories!

As I mentioned earlier, I used to think I was "big-boned" and was doomed with my "man hands." But I'm actually small-boned, and my hands are just an anomaly that I now totally embrace! So be careful that you aren't assuming things about yourself that just aren't true, especially if you've always believed something negative that some-body else told you about yourself. And if there is something you can't change about yourself that you don't like, the way I was with my "man hands," then you just have to change your thinking. Find something you love about that quality!

For example, short girls always say things like "In another life, I'll be taller." I say no way! In this life, you've gotta love what you've got! I used to want to be short. I'm not kidding. I wasn't the tall, gangly girl like most models claim they were in school. I was just average/normal/ nothing special. The tiny girls, the ones who were less than five feet tall, were the cute girls, the cheerleaders, the popular girls all the boys seemed to like. I seriously *longed* to be 4'11"! So if you're short—or have freckles, big feet, frizzy hair, a long nose, or big hands like I did . . . or anything else you can't really change—learn to love it! Make the most of it! Celebrate it as one of your *best features!* Short girls are hot (think Eva Longoria and Lea Michele, both 5'2"), freckles are adorable, big feet make you a great runner and swimmer, frizzy hair can be coaxed into gorgeous curls, a long nose is regal, and like I learned, big hands are awesome for palming a basketball or throwing a perfect spiral with a football.

Model Behavior

If you aren't feeling good, just fake laughing and fake smiling because those actions actually make your body release feel-good hormones, and then what you were faking starts to become real! Your body doesn't know the difference, even if your conscious mind does. You can also fake self-confidence, assertiveness, and *not* being shy. The more you teach yourself how to act out or fake the emotional states and physical situations you want, the more they will come true. It's not mystical. It's just moving yourself in the direction you want to go. Go get what you want and the world will oblige, eventually.

And even if you are big-boned, your bone size says nothing about your actual shape or fitness or weight. And anyway, "skinny" isn't the only option. Think about gorgeous curvy stars like Beyoncé, Kim Kardashian, and Jennifer Lopez. They are all superfit, smoking hot, and healthy, with amazing bodies. If any one of them wanted to get really skinny like a fashion model, sure they could, but they'd lose their boobs and their famous booties and that sexy curvaliciousness they proudly strut. These women love their bodies, and I've seen a lot of different studies saying that men prefer curvy women to "fashionable" thin women.

That reminds me of my friend Cheron. Cheron was a model on *Project Runway,* and we met in L.A. backstage at a show for Nordstrom. She is gorgeous! Tall, blonde, great body, beautiful smile . . . I could go on. Anyway, modeling was never easy for her, and she never seemed happy while doing it. She was good at it, but it just didn't feel like "her." I saw her the other day when I was out with some friends, and I found out she had left modeling and landed a new job.

She was beaming! She asked me how the book was going, and then immediately asked me to guess how much she weighed. This isn't something I tend to think about and I'm not good at it, but she spoke so eagerly that I assumed it must be a positive weight for her. "I can't really tell, but you look great," I said. "Why?"

She gave me this huge smile, and could barely contain herself when she told me that she weighed *more than 140.* I had to laugh because that's still really slim for a girl who is 5'10"—and I also had to laugh with her because *she* laughed and she was just so happy! I could tell she was trying to shock me with the number. She told me she'd never been more toned in her life, and that since she'd quit modeling and gained weight and had been working out a lot, she felt so great—sexy and curvy like a woman. She went on about how in the runway-modeling world, she would be considered too big or too athletic-looking now, but she was stunningly beautiful! She didn't care about the number on the scale. She was happy! And she felt great! This is what every woman's goal should be—to be at the weight that makes you happy and makes you feel sexy, gorgeous, and amazing.

So forget about reaching some ideal that's not you. Maybe you aren't meant to be a size 2/4 or 115 pounds, and so what? Instead, think about how to maximize your own beautiful gifts! Or maybe you are a girl who feels best being superskinny (but *skealthy*— skinny and healthy). And that's great, too. This isn't about someone else. This is about *you,* and self-awareness will help you see what that really means.

So to get all of this straight in your head, I want you to do just three little things:

1. Mirror work

2. Number analysis

3. Q&A with yourself

SUPERMODEL **SAYS . . .**

I think for any individual to feel stronger, prettier, more confident, she must first feel good. Not purely aesthetic, but more like a physiological approach. You must not feel weak, tired, or sick. And the best way to do that is to take care of your body—have a great balance of rest, the right diet, and exercise. If you feel healthy and good about yourself, feeling extra-beautiful should come easily to you. Being a good, happy, helpful person should also help. If you see someone in need, lend a hand. Like if you see a family trying to have a group picture, offer to take their picture. You will feel good after that. Smile and you will get a smile back. Smiling is always positive, and it makes people happy. Lastly, you have to believe in yourself. If you do, you will attract the people around you to believe in you.

— Tutay Maristela-Fasano (aka "2tay"),
flippin' amazing Filipina supermodel

Mirror Work

When I look in the mirror, I know what I want to see from my-self—and myself alone. That wasn't always the case. My grandma still likes to bring up how when I was 12, I hated to go swimming, because I didn't want anyone to see me in a swimsuit. I didn't even want to see myself in a swimsuit! I always wore a T-shirt over my bathing suit, and I even went so far as to forge a doctor's note to get me out of swim class. I made up that I was allergic to chlorine! Talk about lack of confidence. But like the old me, a lot of girls never seem to look at their bodies—*really* look at themselves. They don't want to know how they really look. Being a model has made me more aware of my body, and with that awareness, I've gained a lot of body confidence and the ability to be objective about my own physique.

When I'm checking out my bod in the mirror, I want to see the shape that reflects who I want to be and how I've looked in the past when I felt my best (physically *and* mentally). If I've been stressed or eating poorly or not making time to modercize, I notice that I'm bloated or not as toned as I prefer (and because I have self-awareness, I usually know why!). When I see less definition in my abs or butt, it pisses me off and makes me take action! But I need these little checkups, and I wouldn't be able to see what's going on with my body if I didn't use that mirror. The mirror can help you set your goals and monitor your progress, and once you get *your* supermodel dream body, it can help you keep it.

I never thought I'd be the kind of person who would sit in front of the mirror and stare at myself. I mean, how vain is that? But you don't have to sit there asking if you're the fairest of them all. That's no way to cultivate self-awareness. Instead, you can use the mirror to get to know yourself better.

If you're down on your body, like most girls, try these little tricks. First, everyone looks way hotter in candlelight or dimmed lights, so set the mood! Second, turn on your favorite music, dance, make sexy moves in the mirror—whatever you need to make yourself more comfortable with being naked. Then, really look! Focus on what you love, and where you would like to make some improvements. Try to do this objectively. Don't get all upset with yourself or get caught up in that *How did I ever let myself get this way?* mentality, because that won't help you. That will just make you want to go eat more and forget about the whole thing. Instead, look at yourself with love and compassion. Your body has tried really hard to keep you going, and you need to love it and take care of it so it can feel its best. Look at yourself like that.

You might be thinking, *Well, sure, you're a model—of course you're comfortable being naked.* That's true, finally, after dealing with it for years, because models are always half-naked in front of people. But at first, I was extremely shy and embarrassed, and I hated that part of it—getting undressed with others around and having other people dress me. Eventually, I lost that inhibition because I had to, but it doesn't mean I lost all my insecurities. I have them, too. All models do! For example, I hate wearing thongs. I think they make my butt look ugly and dimply, but for a model, a nude thong is the uniform. We all have a million pairs of them because nobody in fashion wants to see panty lines or any hint of underwear that might distract from the fashion. Sometimes, they even tell us to go commando. Yep, no panties allowed. Weird, I know. One of the ways I learned to cope with it was by using the mirror. I figured out which styles of thongs flattered my bum the best, and how to stand so I always put my best cheek forward!

When I don't like my reflection, I have a heart-to-heart with myself and go through why I'm feeling that way. Sometimes I even talk to myself out loud! Dorky, but totally true, and it works because it helps me focus on what's really going on with me, and that's how I get motivated to get back on track and back into balance with the Five Keys.

Model Behavior

Nothing gives you a self-awareness reality check like seeing a picture of yourself! Models spend most of their time in front of the camera (when they're not sitting around waiting for shoots to start). But even if posing isn't your profession, you still want to look great in your video blog, Instagram and Facebook posts, or profile on a dating site. Who *doesn't* want to look good in pictures, even if it's just from a girls' night out, your mom's birthday party, or a vacation with your family?

When you know how to pose for pictures and look pretty, you can stop deleting so many photos of yourself (you know how that goes: *delete, delete, oh god . . . delete!!!*). Posing well for a photo takes self-awareness. Here are some tips:

- Don't forget your model posture! If you're being shot from the front, push your tush back so your legs will look superskinny and longer. I'm not exaggerating. Try it! Stand in the mirror (naked or in lingerie or a bikini) and strike a pose and notice your thighs. Now, stand up straight (posture!) and push your butt up and back. Look how much thinner your thighs look! It might seem like this position would make your stomach stick out, but it actually draws your stomach back, too. Now try the opposite. Push your butt forward so your hips jut out in front of you. This widens your thighs. Don't do that in the picture!

- Breathe. It relaxes you. Even if you're holding a pose or a facial expression (like a smile), you can still breathe. Remember your beauty breath!

- Find the light and use it to your advantage. The light in the room or the sunlight can show you off and make you look your best. Find it, know where it's coming from, and use it. Lighting is what makes you beautiful, not Photoshop. If you are not lit properly, that's when you get shadows under your eyes, dark roots, and other unattractive illusions. Good lighting can make you look flawless. It brightens you. It beautifies. It makes your entire being light up.

- Feel whatever emotion you want to convey. If it's a fun night with friends, feel like fun. If it's a happy-picture moment, be and feel happy. If it's a sexy one, think sexy. Cute, cute. Excited, excited. Missing someone, miss him or her. And so on. See the eye of the camera as the eye of a person you're trying to convey this feeling to.

- Paying attention to your hands is important, too. Just notice what they're doing.

- Show your face! Most people look best straight on and not to the side.

What if you just really don't feel like having your picture taken? This happens to me sometimes when I don't feel pretty or I'm just not in the mood. That's when I cross my eyes, stick out my tongue, or make some other silly face. It's fun, funny, and being true to my emotions that are telling me there's no pressure to look good at this moment! It can get annoying feeling like you always have to look good in photos.

But back to being naked—you don't have to be naked in front of anybody if you don't want to be. This is just between you and your supermodel self. Just give yourself a frank look because you learn a lot from the mirror. Look at your overall shape. Are you one of those straight-up-and-down, rectangular girls without hips? Are you more like an inverted triangle, with your shoulders broader than your hips? Or more pyramid-shaped, with your hips broader than your shoulders? Or more hourglass-shaped, with your hips and shoulders both broad and a small waist? Whatever your shape, you can rock it. You can look great and feel great. But you need to see what you are so you can love it and maximize it. You might have killer legs or awesome arms or slammin' curves, or you might be elegant and willowy—or you might have the potential to have any of these things. When you see it, you can get there. But you have to see it first. See what looks great, and see where you'd like to make some adjustments.

Using the mirror can also help you refine how you actually want to appear. For models, it's a professional exercise! One of the first things my modeling agency recommended to me in order to learn how to pose and see what looks good was to use the mirror regularly. Despite this truly brilliant advice, I didn't adopt staring into the mirror and posing for quite some time. I was and am in many ways the anti-model, and okay, maybe I'm a little bit rebellious.

But eventually I came around! I've recently embraced the power of the mirror. You can convince yourself of a lot of things, but the mirror doesn't lie. (Although there is this fat mirror in my gym that makes me look so wide and stubby—I know I'm not, but I hope other girls don't see themselves in that mirror and get discouraged! They might as well put one of those funhouse mirrors in the locker room . . . *sheesh!* Or maybe that would be a good idea, to make everybody laugh!) Use the mirror to your advantage! (Okay, you can put your clothes back on now.)

You can also learn a lot about your face from the mirror. I realized, after a lot of mirror "reflection," that I have a slightly crooked mouth, which perfectly matches my slightly crooked teeth. And you know what? I love this about myself! You can see exactly what you look like when you smile, when you frown, when you slouch. How do you look when you're concentrating, or laughing full-out with your mouth open? At first, too much mirror time might make you overly self-conscious in a bad way, especially if you didn't realize you looked like *that* when you got angry or when you were smiling. It can make you feel self-critical. But that's not what we're going for here. We're refining your self-awareness!

SUPERMODEL **SAYS . . .**

Focus on what you really want, and try to make your dreams come true because anything and everything is possible. When I first started modeling and didn't really know how to pose, someone told me to practice my poses in front of a mirror. I tried it and it showed me better ways to sit, where to put my arms and hands, and how to make my neck longer.

— Veronica Jacques, beautiful Latina model, represented by Wilhelmina Models, New York

Using the mirror can help you make slight adjustments to your smile, your frown, your serious look, your happy look. It can help you see that you aren't standing as straight as you could be, and it can help you look better when you walk, because you can see where you're going wrong, putting too much weight on one side or turning your foot or whatever. The point is that you're learning how to look the way you want to look, the way *you* feel like looking, not how anybody else thinks you should look. Just try it. Work on it. Study yourself. The mirror doesn't have to be your enemy. It can be the tool you use to become your own BFF. And that's how you start practicing self-love. (Strutting in front of the mirror marveling at your own hotness totally counts as modercizing!)

The other thing the mirror does—aside from helping you to slightly adjust your look, posture, and gait with a practiced eye—is that it gets you *used to how you look.* I can't believe how many girls just glance in the mirror, then look quickly away, or who only look at a single part, like the one eye where they are applying mascara, but never step back and look at their whole selves. Look. Look, look, and look, until you really know who you are looking at. Let yourself notice things, like where you furrow your brow when you concentrate, causing tiny lines to form between your eyebrows. Self-awareness will help you adjust that. Or how you look in the morning—if you wake up with wrinkles, you probably didn't sleep very well. Maybe you need a more supportive pillow, an eye mask, or a better bedtime routine. It all starts with the mirror! It sounds weird and silly, but it's kind of magical, so please try it!

Being self-aware is knowing yourself, and that includes knowing how you look, how you move, how you act. So your smile is crooked? It's cute that way! So you snort when you laugh? You crinkle your nose when you concentrate? You don't really look very angry when you think you're looking angry? You have a weird dimple, or sometimes you space out and look like you're on another planet? *Know it!* Learn it. Fix the things you don't like, like the way you chew only on one side of your mouth or sit crooked at your desk. See it, feel it, and then you can work on adjusting it.

And the stuff you get to know, and decide is cute? Awesome—feel free to love yourself with abandon, including the way you look, now and tomorrow, before and after you achieve your supermodel body. Even love your body-image issues! (We all have them.) Love your love handles, your muffin top, your double chin. Love them so much that they don't need to get so much attention anymore. Love them and yourself so much that they can fade away as your body transforms. That's how you become self-aware. That's how you learn to love *you*.

MODEL **TALK**

The world is a mirror that will give back to us what we bring to it.

— Mastin Kipp, founder of The Daily Love website and a modern-day superman (sign up for your daily love today: **www.thedailylove.com**)

Here are some more tips for refining what you see in the mirror:

— **Have a loving reflectionship.** It's your relationship with your reflection! Whenever you look in the mirror, pretend like you're looking at someone you're in love with. This is actually how some photographers will get models to look a certain way. For example, when I was shooting for the Japanese magazine *Gisele* in Tokyo, the photographer wanted me to have this romantic, coy, "I'm in love," shy, feminine, sexy look, so he told me to think about the person I was in love with or crushing on. That wasn't too hard because I was *so* crushing on this boy at the time! These are some of my favorite pictures because I can recall that emotional state by just looking at them.

— **Talk pretty.** I do this all the time by saying positive stuff to my reflection. I do so wholeheartedly even though it's silly, and I believe in it—just little things, like a glance in the mirror and a "You rock!" or "Hey, sexy!" or "Lookin' good!" I especially do this when my reflection doesn't show me what I want to see. Say it even when you don't feel it! It can be as simple as greeting yourself with a "Good morning, beautiful!" when you wake up. Or posting or writing positive words of affirmation about yourself on your mirror. It's not vain. It's quirky, in a cute way, and it works magic.

— Whenever you look in the mirror, let it remind you to pay attention and be self-aware. Let it be a self-awareness cue. How do you look when you put on your makeup? I mean all of you, not just the one eyelid. How do you look when you brush your teeth? Wash your face? Brush your hair? Just be aware. The more you know and the more you understand, the more compassionate you will be, with yourself and with everyone else, too.

— Tap the power of images by making a dream board. A dream board is like a poster where you put pictures of all the things you love that help you focus on what you want in life. I know you can do this through Pinterest on your iPhone, but I like to make a real one out of cardboard and photos and cutouts from magazines. This is really fun to do—it's like making your own mirror of everything you love and want, but you have to have an emotional connection with the images. Say, for example, you think you want a body like Kim Kardashian's, but when you look at a picture of her, you feel no emotional connection to that picture. That's not going to work. But if you find a photo of a body that looks like the ideal version of your body, and you cut it out and paste on a picture of your face, and it looks good—like you really look that way, and it gets you amped—then *that* can work. I have a picture on my dream board of a model on the beach. Her body looks healthy and toned, and she's superhappy! You can tell in the picture that she's laughing. Seeing this picture makes *me* feel happy and healthy, and I connect with it, so it works for me. It always makes me feel inspired and back in touch with myself.

SUPERMODEL **PLAYLIST**

This is my personal girl-power playlist for when I need to feel strong, powerful, and beautiful:

Pink, "F**kin' Perfect"
Selena Gomez, "Who Says"
Beyoncé, "Run the World (Girls)"
Kellie Pickler, "Don't You Know You're Beautiful"
One Direction, "What Makes You Beautiful"
Christina Aguilera, "Beautiful"
Bruno Mars, "Just the Way You Are"
Katy Perry, "Firework"
Sarah Brightman, "Beautiful"
Lady Gaga, "Born This Way"
Whitney Houston, "I'm Every Woman"
Kelly Clarkson, "What Doesn't Kill You (Stronger)"

Number Analysis

The next step is to get some stats down on paper. Models carry around these cards called comp cards, usually about 5 × 7 inches or a little bigger, that list all their physical attributes. This is so agencies and clients can decide which girls to use. Let's make your very own Supermodel YOU comp card!

Okay, you may or may not like this part, but this is where we get on the scale, break out the measuring tape, and do some assessment about where you are versus where you're going. First, let's talk about the scale—that horrible, dreaded, obsession-inducing scale!

I feel ambivalent about the scale. I get why people fear it and obsess about it. It's a good idea to get on that scale and know how much you weigh. It's all part of self-awareness. But remember the difference between self-awareness and obsession. That's where you need to draw the line and know yourself, because if weighing yourself every day (twice a day?) makes you crazy, you should cut back to once a week or whatever will let you monitor where you are without making you feel like that one number is going to make or break your whole day.

The number is just a number—a progress report. If it's higher or lower than you want it to be, then you use the Five Keys to get back into balance, and the number will go back to where you want it. It's not about forcing the number down or up unnaturally. It's about *balance,* so remember that it's just a measure. Maybe you don't like the number you see right now, but think of it as a project.

It's also important to stay flexible. Truthfully, I always thought I wanted to be 125 pounds because I read that Nikki Taylor or some other supermodel was 125 and 5'11". I'm close to 5'11" and I thought she looked amazing, so that was my goal. But my body didn't find its happy balance at 125. My body found its happy balance at 117, and I've never felt physically better in my life. This is how I finally understood what my ideal weight was—it was all about what makes me *feel* the best. Who thought I would actually end up weighing *less* than my goal? Certainly not me.

Another thing you might be concerned about when you weigh yourself is your BMI, or body mass index. This is the way health professionals will often assess whether or not you are at a healthy weight. Using a calculation with your weight and height, it provides a range of weight that you should supposedly fall into if you are healthy. It's a good general way to keep track of your weight, but it's not necessarily going to be accurate for you. It doesn't consider muscle mass or bone size. If your BMI says you're overweight, but you feel great and sexy, then ignore it. Maybe you lift weights a lot and you're totally ripped, or maybe you just feel fantastic with a few more curves. The same goes the other way—when I was in the "normal" range, I didn't feel well or balanced. Now I'm a little bit under, and that feels right for me.

Many models are in the "underweight" zone of BMI, but that doesn't mean they're anorexic or whatever (see Chapter 2). It just means that they have found a personal weight that works for them. As long as you feel good, have energy, aren't missing periods, and look the way it feels right for you to look based on your self-awareness, then a too-high or too-low BMI isn't necessarily an indicator of poor health. According to the BMI calculator, supermodel Gisele Bündchen is underweight, and her husband, NFL quarterback Tom Brady, is bordering on the obese. I don't think so!

Calculate Your BMI—But Don't Necessarily Swear by It

By now you might be wondering what your BMI is, exactly. To calculate it, just divide your weight in pounds by your height in inches squared, then multiply that number by 703. The standard interpretation is that having a BMI less than 18.5 is considered unhealthy and underweight, a BMI ranging from 18.5 to 24.9 is considered healthy, and a BMI ranging from 25 to 29.9 is considered unhealthy and overweight. A BMI of 30 or more is considered obese. So know it, but also know yourself. You are a better judge of your personal health and balance than some math formula.

Actually, models are rarely weighed—it's our measurements that matter more to designers and agents. So maybe I'm not as attached to the scale number as some people. Still, I do think it matters. We all fluctuate two to five pounds on any given day, based on water and other factors, but if you suddenly gain ten pounds, that's a sign that you might want to check in with the Five Keys because there's some kind of imbalance. Or pregnancy! Something is happening, and self-awareness means knowing what it is so you're the one in control of it.

So, about those measurements—measurements are what really matter for a model because they determine which clothes will fit which models. This is why we have those group fittings, with a bunch of models in a room all trying on the outfits. As you work with the Five Keys and get back into balance, you'll see your measurements change, and that's fun! So take them the way a model does:

- Bust, across the largest part of your breasts

- Waist, at the smallest part

- Hips, at the widest part around your butt

How to Measure Your Supermodel Self

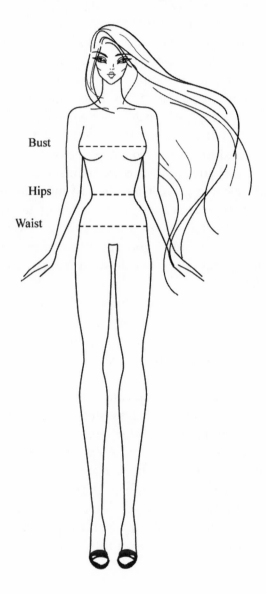

Bust

Hips

Waist

Most models aim for the ideal of 34/24/34, but they rarely hit that mark, despite what you might have read. Most models are probably closer to 34/26/37 or even bigger. So have a goal, but keep in mind that how you feel is the most important part.

Your measurements can also give you more specific info about your body type. When your bust, waist, and hips are all pretty close, like your waist is within six inches of your bust and hips, you're probably a rectangle. If your bust is more than three inches larger than your hips, you're an inverted triangle. If your hips are more than three inches larger than your bust, you are a pyramid. If your bust and hips are about the same (within three inches of each other), and your waist is more than six inches smaller than both, you're an hourglass. These are just my silly shape words to describe body types, not anything to make you feel bad about *your* shape. As I said before, every single shape can look awesome and sexy as long as you are in good health, you modercize, you eat well, you get enough sleep, you de-stress regularly, and you stay in energy balance.

When you put all of this together, you'll have a picture in your mind and some numbers in your head, and that can all flow together with your energy balancing and keeping the Five Keys strong. Just don't get too hung up on any one part. Life is full of surprises!

So let's fill out your comp card, where you can keep track of your progress as you refine and master the Five Keys. Use the following format to copy into your journal, so you can track your stats. Update your numbers once a week, as you work through refining and locking down the Five Keys and getting into energy balance. Watch how the numbers change—you're going to love this part! You'll feel so proud of yourself as you see your numbers transform. See what starts to happen to them as you follow the 20-day plan in the last chapter of this book!

My Supermodel YOU Comp Card

I am beautiful. Here's the proof!

Today's date: _____

Today's weight: _____

Today's measurement: _____

Bust: _____

Waist: _____

Hips: _____

This is all about letting the mirror, the scale, and the tape measure be your self-awareness boosters. Just don't let them run the show. Obsession is the dark side of self-awareness, and when you go there, you can get even more out of balance than when you don't sleep or you overeat or get stressed. Above all those tools—which are just tools, only *tools*—how you feel is the most important thing of all.

Model Pretty

Changing your life can feel like hard work, even when it's fun. If you start to get stressed (remember Key 3!), one of the best things you can do is take a long, full, deep beauty breath. I call this a beauty breath because deep breathing actually makes you look better.

Photographers often put wind fans on the models during a photo shoot, especially when a model is stressed or things just aren't working. The fan creates movement in the hair and clothes. It's a great effect, and it helps relax the model and make her feel more beautiful. Whenever this happens to me, it really feels like it changes everything. The wind blows my hair and my clothes, it opens my eyes, and it forces me to breathe in—and suddenly, the whole energy of the shoot changes. You don't need to turn a fan on yourself to light yourself up like this (although you might want to try it—it makes you feel sexy!). But you can get the same effect by taking a few very deep, calming beauty breaths. Pull out that mirror and see how different you look before and after.

Q&A with Yourself

The last thing I want you to do to fully and completely model-ize your life is to get to know yourself by asking and then answering some really important questions. We're going to go back over all of the Five Keys and all of the aspects of your life that you can control, and we're going to make them personal to *you*.

You can just think about the answers to these questions, but I would *love* it if you would write down the answers, because something about writing what you think and feel makes it more real and makes you more aware of it than if it's just a passing thought flitting through your mind. Plus, then you can go back and read it. You could type your answers on your computer or on your phone, or you could go old-school and get a cool journal and actually write your answers *by hand* (I know, *so* last century). Whatever is more likely to make you do it, that's your method.

Key 1: Self-Awareness Q&A

Let's talk about some real-life techniques to tweak your self-awareness. One of my favorite ways I advise people to do this is through their job. No matter what your job is, there are a lot of ways you can use it to understand yourself and to build cues into your day to help you be more self-aware. How do you identify with your job? Models have an advantage with this one. Models identify with themselves as models (that is, tall, thin, beautiful, confident—all those stereotypes). We tell ourselves, *You're a model. You're hot.* And what a difference that makes! Seriously! All people forge their identities through their jobs to some extent, but because a model's job is based on looking hot, we identify with the stereotype—maybe not all of us, but probably most of us, especially since the stereotype is mostly a positive one.

You might not necessarily identify a particular look with your job, but you probably attribute certain other traits to yourself based on your career. Use that to your advantage. No matter what your career or profession is, you can "super-ize" it. A model just getting started could tell herself she is a supermodel. Why not? It's a great confidence boost—fake it 'til you make it! In the same way, a teacher could tell herself she is a supermodel teacher. A writer could identify herself as a supermodel writer. A personal assistant could be a supermodel personal assistant. It works for any career or job—waitress, lawyer, office worker, medical student, musician, mom. Get some modeltude and you can be the supermodel version of that job! Take all the great things you need to do that job and pat yourself on the back big-time for doing them so well. Add the Five Keys and you've modelized yourself!

Describe your job or career. Now think how you fit into that description. Think specifially about how you look and present yourself. Make a list of ways you could tweak your look or attitude. Could you wear those scrubs like they are cute workout clothes? Can you be the most put-together teacher at the school or the most fashion-forward receptionist in the building? Can you take pride in how you look even if you work at home? The point isn't to be uncomfortable or something you're not, but to take pride in every part of yourself so you feel more confident and beautiful. This is how you modelize your job.

Now, let's insert some cues into your workday. Think about a part of your job you do on a regular basis, at least a few times per day, that you could use as a Supermodel YOU cue. Pick something you'll remember, and an aspect of the keys you need to work on, like posture, beauty breathing, or a modercizing moment.

— Do you go to an office every day? Remember every time you walk in the door at work to turn on your supermodel posture: shoulders back, core in, head held high!

— Do you sit at a computer? Every time the phone rings, use the ensuing conversation as an excuse to fidget at your desk or get up and pace—it's modercize!

— Work on the 20th floor? Take three flights up, two flights down, then jog on the elevator. When you're really rocking the modercizing, maybe you'll walk up 10 flights, or 15, or the whole way eventually!

— Students, don't just sit there at the end of every class. Get up, move around, take a walk—your body is begging for it! Walk from class to class as fast as you can while still maintaining your supermodel posture.

— If you work at a cash register, every time you ring up a customer and the drawer opens, check your posture and your weight distribution to be sure you aren't slouching over onto one hip. Keep your weight even and your posture straight, core in, shoulders back. Rock that register!

— Stay-at-home moms and pretty much everyone else who ever has to clean anything, how do you stand while doing dishes? I'm tall and used to find myself hunched over the sink, or leaning more to one side to get closer to the faucet. Now, I spread my legs to shorten myself and make sure my core is in, and then I'm balanced! How do you carry the laundry basket? Off to one hip? How do you carry your child?

Now think of a cue you can use in your own work or in your day, and where you can remind yourself about posture, movement, and just telling yourself you rock. What are your cues, and what are you going to do whenever you get those cues?

Here are some writing prompts for your journal. Try to think of at least three to five.

- Cue: _____
- What it reminds me to do: _____

Now that you've got your cues in place, I want you to think about your life in general. Apart from your job, and in fact apart from *everything* you associate yourself with or that you feel gives you an identity but is external, think about who you are. Try not to think about how other people see you, including your friends, partner, and family. Try not to assign an identity to yourself based on your job, your clothes, your hair, your hobbies, your favorite foods, your favorite songs, your favorite places. Let all of that go, open your journal, and just think about these questions:

- What do you want out of your life?

- Do you feel like you could know yourself better? Where do you feel like you are still somewhat of a mystery to yourself?

- Do you feel differently than you felt as a child? In what ways?

- What parts of yourself do you think you've lost touch with that you used to love?

- What parts of yourself do you think you truly understand?

Describe the supermodel version of you—your best version of yourself.

Now, what's the difference between you and the above description?

The preceding is a list of your projects! The Five Keys are the path between these two separate versions of you. You have the power to become Supermodel YOU! Do you believe it? Here's where you convince yourself. Tell yourself how awesome you are!

Key 2: Beauty Sleep Q&A

You know by now all the things you *should* do to get a good night's sleep, but let's look at what you're *actually* doing, and how you can make some real changes for better ZZZs. Here are some practical applications. Let's talk about your sleep habits!

- How well do you sleep? How would you describe your sleep quality?

- How many hours of sleep do you get on average during the week?

- How many hours of sleep do you get on average during the weekend?

- Do you nap? Are you able to nap, or even just close your eyes and turn off your brain for a while?

- What things make you automatically feel sleepy that you might be able to integrate into your sleep regimen (like music, low lights, a hot bath, certain foods, a sleep mask, lavender oil, or any of the other suggestions from the sleep chapter).

- What sleep robbers tend to deprive you of your ZZZs (like too much liquid before bed, alcohol, loud music, television and computer time, exercising at night, and so on)?

Make a sleep plan, based on eliminating sleep robbers and adding sleep enhancers. Every night before you go to bed (or whenever possible), follow this plan for the ultimate snoozefest.

Key 3: De-stressing Q&A

Everybody gets stressed-out sometimes, but for a lot of us, it's a chronic problem, and *so* not pretty! It's time to get a handle on your stress.

- What stresses you the most? Make a list of your ten biggest stressors.

- What de-stresses you? What are the top ten things that totally relax, calm, and balance you (even if you don't get to do them all that often)?

- Look back over the stress chapter. How could you start to reduce some of your worst stressors? What model tips might apply to you?

Pick one thing you can do every time you notice you are feeling stressed, like fidgeting, taking a big beauty breath, going for a walk, assuming a yoga position, or just taking a few minutes of quiet time to close your eyes and relax (in a word, to *meditate*). Practice doing it as often as you need it. What will your one stress antidote be? (You can totally change it from week to week.)

Key 4: Modercizing Q&A

Let's start with your posture, because not only is it so important to how you look and feel, but good posture also burns way more calories than slumping. So let's pay attention to your posture for a minute.

Do you have any idea how your posture looks right now? Think about it. Slouch for a second. (Or maybe, like most people, you already are.) Now slouch even more. How do you feel? Do you feel fat or skinny? Confident or embarrassed? Would you want a bunch of people you didn't know very well to walk into the room and look at you right now, exactly like that, in that slouching position? If you really don't know how bad it looks, do it in front of the mirror.

Now take a breath and sit up straight. Try to be as tall as you can. Feel a lifting from the crown of your head. Roll your shoulders back. Look straight out in front of you.

Now how do you feel? I'll tell you one thing: you *look* way hotter than you did in that sorry slouch.

When you stand up tall, your blood flows more freely, and so does your confidence (a study from Ohio State University found that participants who sat up straight felt more confident). Sitting or standing up straight also makes you appear ten pounds lighter, and it burns more calories than slouching. Not too shabby for a slight physical adjustment!

Body language is superpowerful, and nobody knows this like a model. Models are expected to know how their body language translates on film or the runway. Every move, every glance, every adjustment has to look a certain way, so we're very aware of our posture and gait. It's totally become ingrained in our minds to always walk and carry ourselves a certain way (erect and with a brisk pace). Models strut with confidence in the grocery-store aisle, while walking the dog, and into a café in SoHo to splurge on a skinny latte. Being tall and thin doesn't make everyone look like a model, but I can always spot a real model based on her body language. If you want to look like the supermodel version of yourself, this is what you need to do. Develop confident body language that makes you look and feel sexier: shoulders back, chin up, tummy in.

The more you do this, the more it will become second nature. One good way to ingrain this habit is to create situational triggers for yourself, like checking your posture every time you exit an elevator, open any door in your home, or pass a cute guy on the street (because he might look back at you!). You can use any cue that speaks to you (meaning one that you will actually *use*).

I was doing a fashion show at Busch Gardens in Florida where the models were hired to "turn into" vampires, and whenever the models heard a horn sound, it was our cue to assume our catwalk attitudes and strut our stuff! Every time we heard that noise, it was crazy how "on" we became. In a few moments, we were totally conditioned to ramp up self-awareness so we could turn on the modeltude! Even now, when I hear a horn blow (often in songs on the radio), I instantly turn on the "model-vampire" in me. It's amazing how easily it works to assign a cue to a behavior.

You can totally use this to your benefit! Here are some more ideas for reminding you to turn on the modeltude: What's your favorite song? Every time you hear it, check your posture. Or every time you see your favorite or lucky number, whether it's on a street sign or billboard, make sure your body is in full model stand-up-tall position. If this is all too passive for you, let your phone do the work. Set the alarm to go off at various intervals as a reminder to modelize. Send yourself text messages on a schedule. *New York Times* best-selling author Cheryl Richardson uses the app TellMeLater to remind herself that she is beautiful and amazing. Download it! You can send yourself messages like "Wake up to your beauty!" or "Remember who you are" or "Pay attention!" or "How's your posture?" or "Are you doing what you really want to be doing right now?" or just "You totally rock!" Anything to get your own attention. Pretty soon, you won't even need the reminders anymore.

There are plenty of other ways to "cue up" and modelize your modercize in your life right now. Some ideas:

- Think about how much and in what way you move in your life. How do you get most of your exercise? Walking? Running? Going to the gym? Yoga? Or maybe you really don't exercise at all?

  How could you step up the modercizing? What ideas sound fun to you? Could you walk faster? Lose the heels so you pick up speed? Take the stairs instead of the elevator? Fidget more? Go dancing once a week? Shop more? Kiss more? What's your plan?

- What situations make you feel like moving? Being outside? That gym smell? Incense in a yoga room? Music? List your movement inspirations.

- What do you like to do? Modercizing should be totally fun. Is there a way you could modercize more while doing your favorite things?

- What things make you less likely to get moving? High heels? Cold weather? Uncomfortable clothes? Food comas? (Pay attention to why *that* happened!) Deadlines at the office? Sleeping in? Then list ways you could modify some of these so you modercize on more days than you do now. Make a plan!

Key 5: Intuitive Eating Q&A

People always ask me about how I eat. It's the main thing that affects body weight, so that makes sense. If you're truly self-aware (and all the keys go back to self-awareness), you'll be able to recognize when you're eating because you're actually hungry, as opposed to being bored or stressed-out or just two feet away from a really yummy-looking bag of chocolate-chip cookies.

Food availability is a major temptation, so it's really important *not* to buy food you can't resist, and not to keep it in your house. For example, I can't have coffee in my house, because I will gravitate toward it and I don't want to be addicted to anything. Then, when I do occasionally have coffee at a restaurant or a job, I appreciate it so much more! And I drink it with more self-awareness. I actually asked my dad to take the coffeemaker out of the house so I wouldn't be tempted—out of sight, out of mind. It worked like magic.

Nerd Alert!

Some health professionals believe that the very foods we crave the most are the ones that aren't good for us. I go crazy for mushrooms. I could eat hundreds of them. It's the same with peanut butter. Get it out of my sight! I will devour the entire jar in one sitting! But guess what? I'm *allergic* to both mushrooms and peanut butter! Not the deathly ill kind of allergic, but I have intolerances to both of these foods, and a lot of others, like nuts and broccoli. Yes, broccoli! I learned all this through a hair-analysis test, and this test changed my life because I realized how many foods were keeping me from feeling my best, interfering with my sleep, and messing with my digestion.

I encourage you to get one of these tests if you want to see what foods might be secretly stressing out your hot bod. It costs $175, but I worked out a *Supermodel YOU* reader discount, so check out the company's website. You will get the test for $125, along with a 10 percent discount on supplement orders, as long as you use the code "Supermodel." Find out more here: **www.rumiom.com/index.php/ hair-kit/order-a-hair-analysis.html**.

A Cornell University study found that college secretaries ate twice as many Hershey's Kisses when they were placed on their desk than when they were placed six feet away. The secretaries also lost track of how many they had eaten when they didn't have to move to get to the food. This is a sure sign that self-awareness has lapsed. If you're aware of eating, you'll know exactly how much you've eaten, even if you didn't measure it. You'll never eat automatically, mindlessly. Your mind will be engaged in eating, as it should be. It's the only way to really, truly eat what you need.

I talked about all of this in the intuitive-eating chapter, but I just want to remind you that eating is all about knowing yourself and knowing what you are likely to do. I was walking to the car with a model friend after a runway show one evening, and she had this bag of mixed nuts. She opened it up, looked at it, and offered me some, and when I didn't want any, she threw the bag into the garbage. Why waste the food? Well, she realized she wasn't actually hungry, but she also knew herself well enough to know that she would dig in to those nuts just because she could.

I've often heard of celebrities doing this—like taking one bite of dessert and then pouring water on it, or ruining it in some other way. It's self-awareness at work, even if it seems strange to someone who wouldn't have trouble saying no to something sweet. Self-awareness means knowing what you are likely to do, even if it's not what you *should* do. Self-awareness isn't about pretending to be perfect. It's about acknowledging and accepting imperfections.

So let's look at you and how you eat. One of the very best, most powerful ways to apply self-awareness to your eating is to keep a food diary, at least for a while. There are tons of good apps for this (I'm working on one myself!) that will tell you the caloric and nutritional content of what you eat, making food diaries supereasy. I highly recommend doing this. It's not about being obsessive. It's about being aware, rather than being in denial about how much you're actually eating.

Also, answer these questions to tune you in even more to your habits, preferences, and tendencies:

- What are your food weaknesses—the things you know you will overeat if they are available? (Mine are fried plantains and sweet potatoes—weird, right?)

- When you get a food craving, what else are you feeling? The next time you get one, really try to notice and pinpoint the accompanying feeling. Is it anxiety? Boredom? Depression? Feeling hyperactive? PMS?

- Are you drinking enough water? How much water do you drink on most days? How much water did you drink so far today?

SUPERMODEL **SAYS . . .**

I prefer to eat my calories, not drink them. Stay away from fruit juice, soda, and specialty coffee drinks. If you must, have a simple espresso, and drink lots of water! Water flushes out everything. It's a youth and diet elixir. I drink two liters a day, and I always carry a one-liter bottle in my bag wherever I go, for easy access.

— Cynthia Kirchner, beauty and lingerie model, known for her bangin' body, beautiful hair, and perfect skin

Think of three substitutes that would be healthier versions of the top three unhealthy foods you tend to crave. For instance, I hardly ever see models eating candy bars, but I often see them eating protein bars, which are basically like fortified candy bars, with added protein and vitamins. Other examples might be to substitute fresh fruit when you have a craving for candy, Greek yogurt when you have a craving for ice cream, or unbuttered popcorn or celery and carrots when you have a craving for chips. Use the following template to help you match your unhealthy cravings to healthier options in your journal.

- Unhealthy food craving: _____
- Substitute #1: _____
- Substitute #2: _____
- Substitute #3: _____

Now consider these additional questions and ideas:

- What situations make you most likely to overeat? (Like social gatherings, parties, restaurants, or when you're home alone and nobody's watching?)
- What could you do during those trigger situations that would fill up your desire to overeat? (Make the effort to join a conversation at a party, or start

dancing? Order only an appetizer at a restaurant, or split an entrée? Or when you're home, go for a walk, call a friend, put on your favorite music, or take a bath?) Write some trigger-situation solutions in your journal.

- Get trigger food out of your house. Out of sight, out of mind! Out of your cupboard, fridge, freezer, and off your frickin' property! This is what I have to do with coffee and peanut butter. Let's say ice cream is your weakness. Don't keep it in the house! Instead, only have it when you walk (modercize) to an ice-cream shop for a special treat once in a while. Walking to the ice-cream shop burns a lot more calories than walking to your fridge. What trigger foods do you need to get out of sight, out of mind? Make a list of five or more in your journal.

- Try eating pretty. Pay attention to each bite, chew carefully with your mouth closed, even watch yourself eat in a mirror. Try using smaller plates and utensils. Be dainty. (Remember the Rule of the Fist— that's all the room you have in your stomach, so why use a giant plate?) Describe how that felt in your journal.

- How do you feel about the way you eat? What do you do right, and what are you going to work on? Use your journal to make a plan for tomorrow.

■ ■

The whole point of modelizing your life is to take everything you've learned from this book and make it about *you*. You are the supermodel of your own life. We are all totally different, and you can imitate some of what models do, but in the end, it's really about self-awareness. It's the most important part of all. It's what this whole book is really about. Master that, and you're beautiful, no matter what stage of progress you've achieved. It's self-awareness that makes Supermodel YOU, so let it be about *you*. Because it really is.

■ ■ ■

CHAPTER TEN

Supermodel YOU in Action!

I think it's very important never to compare yourself to another person. The worst thing you can do to yourself is beat yourself up because you don't have what someone else has. That said, as my mother taught me from an early age, it's also not great to think of yourself as better than others. As a model, I like to think of myself as a blank canvas that artists and stylists get to embellish into something amazing. I think everyone can be like that. Make yourself the canvas. Embellish yourself with a beautiful personality and it will radiate from within. I truly do believe that beauty from within will always make you feel more beautiful in general.

— Stefanie Wood, superchef and model,
represented by PhotoGenics

"Runway, lights, model, *go!*" This is the cue models get at the start of a fashion show, and if you're the first girl out, the girl who opens the show, you will generally get a little push right on the "go." This chapter is your push! It's your cue to hit the runway of your life and start making the real changes you need in order to truly succeed as Supermodel YOU: gorgeous, stunning, happy, confident, sexy *you!* This is your life, and life is your runway. It's what you make of it.

Don't worry if you trip and fall, or slip up. Almost every single model has fallen at one time or another. Models have fallen flat on their faces. Life is full of crazy falls and unexpected disasters, but a good model always gets back up and keeps going. We have to! If you want to realize your dream body, dream career, and dream life, you can't let momentary setbacks stop your progress. I promise that when you have the Five Keys in check, you will have your life, body, and health in check as well. You can't get very far down the road if you lose your car keys, and you can't unlock the front door if you've misplaced your house keys—and it's no different with the *Five Keys*. The keys to Supermodel YOU are the keys to your best life—the life you've always wanted and the one you know you deserve.

You become what you repeatedly do, and if the average work/schoolday is eight hours, then eight hours a day you are becoming what you do. It's time to apply the Five Keys of Supermodel YOU to what you do most of the time. Almost every day, you tie your shoes, brush your teeth, shower, open the fridge, get out of bed, walk in and out of the same doorway, hear certain sounds, and see certain things. Adding a trigger cue to these tasks will help you check in with the Five Keys.

For instance, every time I open the fridge, I check in with myself and see if I'm truly hungry or doing this out of habit. Every time I hear the phone ring, I remember my supermodel posture and take a beauty breath. By anchoring these seemingly insignificant gestures to things you do and see almost unconsciously, you will begin to reprogram the way you think, act, eat, and move. By doing this even just a few times, you will start to reprogram your life in a way that will become second nature.

But maybe you want more structure? If you like to follow a plan and you want some help integrating the Five Keys into your life, this is your chapter. It's time to make over your life, one key and one step at a time.

Remember when I told you that studies show it takes 20 days to form a habit? I'm going to give you 20 days to make over your life. Each day, you'll get a new strategy for integrating one of the Five Keys into your life. By the end of 20 days, it will be a whole new you—a Supermodel YOU! Then just keep going at your own pace. And remember: You are no longer a nurse, a teacher, an assistant, a stay-at-home mom, or whatever role you identify with. You are now a supermodel nurse, a supermodel teacher, a supermodel assistant, a supermodel mom, and so on! This is part of your new job description. You don't have to announce it to the world, but you must remind yourself every day: "I am *super*. I can be anything I want to be." Wake up every day and say to yourself, "Good morning, Supermodel ME!" Right before bed, say to yourself, "Sweet dreams, beautiful Supermodel ME!" And mean it!

Are you ready to change your habits, change your life, and start living like a supermodel? Runway, lights, Supermodel YOU, *go!*

Day 1

The first four days are all about Key 1: self-awareness. Today, you are going to create triggers for posture while you're at work. Upon entering your job, whenever you see X co-worker, punch into the time clock, open a drawer, or whatever it is you do frequently throughout the day, anchor your posture awareness with one or two tasks. Whenever you do, see, hear, or experience those triggers, pull your shoulders back, hold in your core, straighten your spine, look out boldly at the world, and breathe. Think: *I am a supermodel*. Notice how different you feel each time you cue your self-awareness by physically adjusting your posture.

Day 2

Today, you're going to create a modeltude trigger. You're still working on your posture trigger, but this is an *attitude* adjustment. This trigger will remind you to embrace the positive and dump the negative. Create a text alert or an alarm on your phone or computer that repeats several times every day, reminding you that you are gorgeous, amazing, and smokin' hot. Feel it, know it, believe it! Remember that to change your body and your life, you must change your attitude.

Day 3

Today, we're still working on self-awareness, but we're going to apply it to the practical side of your life. Start a new routine: planning for tomorrow. Before you go to bed tonight, check the weather, set out your clothes, prepare any healthy meals or snacks you'll need to take with you in the morning, and decide what time to turn in. No distractions! Follow through with your plan.

Day 4

Today is our last day to concentrate on Key 1, self-awareness. Keep practicing your model posture and modeltude—are your triggers working? Are you developing new habits? Also, maintain your evening routine so you'll always be ready to face each new day. Today, add one more self-awareness strategy: make a commitment to change one (just one!) work-related behavior that you do not feel is creating a positive relationship with you and your body. Are you unnecessarily consuming calories in the form of beverages or food? Are you dipping into that candy jar? Are you taking the elevator instead of the stairs? Or pick something that will improve your mental health. Are you wasting time mindlessly browsing the Internet? Do you always arrive at work a little bit late? Are you gossiping? Are you putting yourself down in your own mind? Spending too much time around negative co-workers? Whatever behavior you choose, it's time to ditch it and move on to brighter habits and mind-sets. Over the next 20 days, you are so over doing that!

Day 5

For the next four days, we'll be tackling Key 2: beauty sleep! You won't forget about Key 1, of course, but today, it's time to prioritiZZZe your sleep. Set a sleep schedule for yourself. Base it on your current schedule. If it's not realistic and doesn't work in your life, you'll never do it (self-awareness will keep you honest). Squeeze in at least seven and a half hours, preferably eight or nine. The more you sleep, the better you will look and feel. Plus, sleep deprivation can make you binge on sweets. No supermodel needs that kind of temptation!

Day 6

Today, you're going to stick to that sleep schedule you set up yesterday, but you're also going to "pimp" your sleep space. First, clean. (Cleaning is a great calorie torcher!) Change your sheets, vacuum, dust, and clear off that cluttered bedside table. Fold the piles of laundry and get anything that isn't related to sleep or sex *o-u-t*. This is your sanctuary, not your home office, or worse, your dumping ground for the junk you don't want anywhere else. You can work on this a little bit at a time all week if you like, or just dive in and do it all.

Now, part two of today's assignment: go shopping. Yes! It's required! *You must shop.* Invest in earplugs or an eye mask to maximize your sleep. Not everybody has blackout curtains in their bedroom, but you need total darkness and quiet to get truly rejuvenating beauty sleep. Do you need anything else? A better pillow? Comfy new sheets? Whatever it is, get what you need (within your budget) so you'll look forward to curling up in bed at night. While you're at it, you might as well start a new-mattress fund. Start saving your pennies! A really good mattress will make you feel super in the morning.

Day 7

Today is the third day of working on Key 2, beauty sleep, and it's time to ritualiZZZe. Devise a sleep ritual to fit into your new sleep schedule—a thing or series of things you will do every night to get your mind and hot bod ready to snooze. Here are some ideas:

- Dim all the lights about 30 minutes before bed.
- Prep your breakfast for the next day.
- Light candles.
- Play relaxing music (no death metal, please—save that for the morning!).
- Take a hot bath, maybe with a few drops of lavender oil.
- Meditate—it's good for your brain! Or pray, if that's more your speed.
- Read a good book.

Once your sleep ritual is a habit, just starting it will begin to make you feel sleepy . . . like you could . . . just . . . drift off. . . .

Day 8

Today is our last superfocused Key 2 day, and this is the day to totally banish sleep robberZZZ. That means no sugar, fatty food, caffeine, or alcohol within one hour of your regularly scheduled bedtime. Now that you've got your schedule and your ritual, you don't need that stuff anyway! Use your DVR to record your shows if they're on late, and turn off the TV or computer. Just say no to anything that gets you too stimulated. (I know I said sex is a stimulant, but if it really does relax you, then you have my permission to get busy.) No dealing with work issues, no fighting with family members or friends. Before bed, everything should be calm, sweet, and sleepy. Set your alarm for the latest possible time to ensure maximum beauty sleep (rather than hitting the snooze button a bunch of times—you know who you are!). Make sure that everything is ready for the morning so that you don't have any pressing thoughts keeping you awake. Sleep robberZZZ are *out!* Sweet dreams! (And you're going to look awesome tomorrow morning!)

Day 9

Today is the first day for Key 3: de-stressing. Although you're probably feeling less stressed already because you're getting so much beauty sleep and you're more self-aware, it's time to institute some specific stress-defying strategies.

Today, identify one aspect of your life that is a major stressor that you can do something about. Now don't get all stressed about what stressor to de-stress—just pick one. One little thing can make a huge difference in your day. Maybe it's that you're always late. Make a plan to start getting ready 30 minutes earlier. Commit to being on time. Models can't afford to be late, and neither can you!

Maybe it's that mornings are such a rush. Remember to get everything ready the night before as part of your bedtime ritual, as you began practicing on Day 3. If it's your job that is too stressful, schedule in mini-meditation or beauty-breath breaks at work, and think about how to reframe your attitude. Or maybe it's something totally different. You pick—whatever you can handle and solve *today.*

Remember: stress is *in your head.* It's all about perception. Change your perception about the thing that stresses you the most, and even without anything else changing—*poof!*—the stress can dissolve, just like that. It's pretty cool.

Day 10

Today, you're going to get rid of stupid stress. Stupid stress is the stress you have total control over, yet you still let get to you. Examples of stupid stress are being late, clenching your fists or jaw, frowning or furrowing your brow (both form wrinkles, so stop it!), wearing uncomfortable clothes that don't fit properly, or making bad food choices that make you feel gross. You exacerbate stupid stress when you slump, carry your purse with one shoulder too high or low, grip the steering wheel too tightly, type on the keyboard with your head jutted forward (stressing your neck), or squinting when you read.

Pick one area of stupid stress and stop being stupid! Remember, models are smarter than people think, and you are smarter than stupid stress. Get it out of your life by deciding to be on time; unclenching your face and fists, and taking a big beauty breath instead; ditching your uncomfortable, ill-fitting clothes and finding killer deals on outfits that actually fit and flatter you; and choosing the foods you know will make you feel rockin'. As you go through your day, think about the ways you're stressing yourself for no reason, and begin to be more self-aware about them so you can *stop doing them!* Eventually you can get rid of *all* your stupid stress. I know you can! But don't worry about doing it all at once. Start with one instance—today is the day you *begin* banishing stupid stress from your life.

Day 11

Today, it's time to take a good, hard look at the people in your life. You know how some people make you feel really great, calm, happy, or confident, while other people make you feel anxious or negative, or encourage you to do things that you regret later? Some people are just too hard to be around. They contribute to stress. They might be Negative Nancys or Vampire Valindas who suck your energy or who are all take and no give. We all have these people in our lives, and we've all been these people at some point in our lives, too—people who are under a lot of stress themselves can be stressful to others. However, now that you are on the path to Supermodel YOU, these individuals will only bring you down. Surround yourself with positive people who make you feel good—with other supermodels-in-spirit, with people who boost your confidence, and with people who have the good habits and healthy lifestyle you want to have. In fact, while you're at it, you might as well just create your own modeltourage—because you become like the company you keep.

Day 12

You're going to love today because it's the day when you are *required* to pamper yourself. A little self-indulgence (the healthy kind, not the kind involving tequila shots or cupcakes) goes a long way toward dissolving the stress that holds you back from your dreams. So get a massage, take a long bath, get a mani/pedi, or do something else just for *you* that you love and that totally relaxes you. This is a day of self-love. Bask in it! (Repeat daily—or at least weekly!)

Day 13

Today we begin tackling Key 4: modercizing. Remember, modercizing doesn't have to be formal exercise. It's just about getting more movement into your daily life in ways that are natural and fun. So today, I want you to dress for modercizing! Wear flats or comfortable shoes (no heels allowed!). No tight, short skirts today. Wear something you can really move in. If you wear reds or oranges, you get bonus points for energizing colors! Use your self-awareness to notice opportunities for walking more, taking the stairs more often, picking up your pace, or just fidgeting when you have to sit or stand for a while. See how much easier it is when your clothes and shoes are made to move?

Day 14

Okay, cleaning lady, today is your day! It's time to clean house, organize your living space, vacuum, dust, scrub the tub, mop the kitchen floor, clean out your closet—whatever needs to be done. Do it with high energy and motivation. Your house or apartment or room is going to look *so much better,* and so will you, because cleaning and de-cluttering burn calories.

Day 15

Today, I want you to make a vow: you will not sit in one place for more than 15 minutes at a time. I'm serious! Even if you have to sit for a prolonged period, get up and walk around, do a few jumping jacks or stretches or yoga poses, and shake off the sedentary! Then you can sit back down and get back to what you were doing. Sitting too much is bad for your bod, so break it up as much as possible. Watching TV counts, too. Intersperse your couch-potato session with sit-ups, push-ups, stair sets, or whatever it is. No more than 15 minutes! I mean it, Supermodel YOU!

Day 16

Today is our last day to focus on Key 4, modercizing, and we're going to make the most of it by fidgeting. Yes! Fidget today. Tap your foot. Bop to your inner groove, or put on your headphones and get funky while you're walking around through your day. Put a spring in your step. Shift in your seat. Get up frequently and jump up and down. Be one of those people who *can't sit still.* Keep it up all day and I guarantee you will be thinner tomorrow.

Day 17

It's finally time for Key 5! You've been waiting for this one, haven't you? Intuitive eating sounds easy, but it's actually challenging . . . *unless* you've got the other four keys in place, which you now totally do, so hooray for you! You're ready to get that crazy sweet tooth or fat tooth or whatever tooth you have under control. Let's start with the basics. Today, I want you to question your appetites. You don't necessarily have to deny them, but I want you to *question* them, using your self-awareness. When you crave something, before you shove it in your mouth, stop, take a beauty breath, and ask yourself: *Is this what I'm really hungry for?* Maybe it is and maybe it isn't, but you'll never know if you don't ask yourself the question, and I mean every single time. No more mindless eating! It's all about awareness now, baby.

Another really great way to stay aware of your food and to question how badly you really want something is to start writing down every single thing you eat and drink. Yes, everything. Even that one brownie bite, even those three chips you stole from your roommate. Question your appetite and record your responses. Are you really hungry when you smell that doughnut? Or is it something else? Be aware of your own body and hunger signals today so that you can learn to tell the difference between fake and real hunger.

Day 18

Today, I want you to do two things: (1) eat a good breakfast, including protein and whole grains; and (2) take the three model must-haves with you when you go out—water, a cell phone, and *snacks!* Put healthy snacks in your purse or car so you aren't tempted to eat junk food when you get hungry later. These two habits—eating a good breakfast and healthy snacks—can make a huge difference in how well you're able to exercise your so-called self-control. It's all about convenience!

Some ideas for breakfast:

- Whole-grain toast with peanut butter and a banana
- Oatmeal with walnuts, blueberries, and cinnamon
- Smoothie with fresh fruit, a handful of leafy greens, and a good-quality protein powder
- Egg-white omelette with lots of veggies

Some ideas for snacks:

- Low-sugar, high-protein bars or fruit/nut bars

- An apple, a pear, or other packable fruit
- Little packets of raw nuts or trail mix
- Bag of fresh veggies cut to bite-size and a container of hummus

And don't forget your bottle of water!

Day 19

Today, it's all about eating pretty. Every single time you reach for a fork or a cup—meals, snacks, slurping your latte—I want you to do it "pretty." Take small, dainty bites and delicate sips. Sit up straight and maintain your model posture while you eat. Handle your utensils gracefully. Stay totally aware of what you are eating—"mindless" is not pretty! Chew quietly with your mouth closed. Pause between bites in order to be fascinated by your dining companion and charming to the waiter (or the barista or your roommate or whomever). From now on, to eat means to look pretty. End of discussion!

Day 20

It's the very last day of your 20-day Supermodel YOU makeover! Can you believe how far you've come? You're self-aware, you're getting enough sleep, you're moving more, you're de-stressing, and you look awesome, even when you're chowing down. On this final day, I want you to consider something extremely important: *What are you putting in your mouth?*

Everybody can make their own decisions about what they do and don't want to eat, but what I would like you to consider today—and for the rest of your life—is not just the quantity of food you eat, but the quality and the content. Do you really want to put fatty meat and cheese, toxic sugar, or chemicals into your fabulous and gorgeous supermodel body? Maybe sometimes you do, but think about how often, and the price of a few minutes of yum. Remember, changing your attitude can change your life. When you decide that you only deserve nutrient-dense vegetables; whole grains; lean protein; juicy fruits; and healthy fats like the kinds that come from nuts, avocados, and coconuts, then that's exactly what you should be eating.

■ ■

Remember, do it for 20 days and it's a habit. You can restart your 20 days whenever you like. If you mess up, so what? You're only human. Just go back to your Supermodel YOU mentality and make a commitment to yourself again.

The final thing I want you to do is to pretend. That's right—start acting like you already have your dream body. Start acting like you already have your dream job, your dream romance, your dream *life*. Pretend you are already perfect, and that everything good and loving and wonderful that you do for yourself is just because you richly *deserve it*.

Pretend it with all your heart. And you know what? It might not be too long before you realize that it's all true.

Whenever you feel like you've fallen off your runway, just check back in with the Five Keys. You didn't sleep well? You're feeling stressed? Feeling a little bit sick, like a cold is coming on? Go back to the keys. Let self-awareness help you see what you're doing that is pushing you off balance. Did you sleep well? Eat well? How's your posture? Have you de-stressed lately? Take a beauty breath and reassess.

And when you are feeling great? Do the same thing to see why you feel so good! Pay attention to how you sleep, eat, stand, move, and think. This is how you start to make good habits second nature.

The Five Keys are the answer, so let them work for you. Stay strong, be kind, live happy, and know how beautiful you really are!

■ ■ ■

AFTERWORD

Models are people, too. Models do a lot of the same things that anybody who wants to get and stay healthy and fit does. They drink lots of juices and smoothies, and eat lots of Greek yogurt, fruit, and vegetables. They move a lot, and many of them do yoga. The difference is that for models, staying fit, healthy, and beautiful is a job requirement.

But models aren't so different from you. They all have their unique personalities, things they love, and things they will never do. They work hard, but not *too* hard. They love music, they need friends, they want love. They're all beautiful, they're all individuals, and they're all *super.* Just like you.

Here, at the end of this book, is the most important thing I want you to remember: let models inspire you, let their *skealthy* habits encourage and motivate you (you'll hear about many of them in Appendix A), but never forget who *you* are. Start with self-awareness and keep on going, because when you truly know who you are and love who you are, then you will become something fantastic, someone better than you ever dreamed—you will become Supermodel YOU.

This book is just the beginning. Let this be the catalyst that helps you open that cocoon. Unfurling your wings and taking off in a gorgeous flight is up to you, but I, for one, can't wait to see what you make of yourself. Because you're a supermodel, in the best possible way—in your *own* way. Happy journey!

xoxo Sarah DeAnna

■ ■ ■

SUPERMODEL YOU
GLOSSARY

Beauty breath: A deep breath that makes you relax and stress less, and reduces facial wrinkles. Always remember to breathe deeply and watch your face change!

Campaign: The whole plan for a company's advertising, including how they will brand their images used for promotion. To be booked for a company's campaign means they will use you in their branding images.

Casting: The audition for a specific job.

Commercial: A classically pretty look, as opposed to an editorial look.

Comp card: A card, usually about 5 × 7 inches, that models carry with them listing all their physical attributes, such as height, weight, measurements, hair color, and eye color.

Editorial: A unique look, as opposed to a commercial look.

FashionSpeak: Definitions of words from the world of modeling.

Go-see: A go-see is like a casting, but not for a specific job. Instead, the model meets the client to show herself off, so the client can decide whether they might like to use her eventually. Go-sees are common with photographers, photographers' agents, and casting directors.

Homeostasis: The tendency of a body (or any system) to maintain a stable equilibrium, such as your body attempting to stay at a particular weight.

Intuitive eating: A way to eat based on your intuition and self-awareness rather than on some external diet plan.

Look: An outfit that a model wears in a photo shoot or a show.

Market: Showrooms set up by designers, often specific to clients and often at the designers' headquarters, that debut collections for buyers from boutiques and department stores. The designers hire models to walk around showing the clothes.

Modelize: To apply model habits and advice to your own life.

Modeltation: The model method of meditation: close your eyes and just go inward, disconnecting yourself from a stressful environment, or focusing on what kind of energy or impression is desired for a photo shoot.

Modeltourage: When a bunch of models all hang out together in public.

Modeltude: The self-confident, *I'm hot* attitude that models tend to have. (See: **www.urbandictionary.com.**)

Modercize: The model version of exercise, which doesn't usually involve the gym, but instead includes nontraditional exercise activities that nevertheless burn calories, such as dancing, cleaning, changing clothes multiple times during work, kissing, shopping, and fidgeting. (See: **www.urbandictionary.com.**)

Mother-agent: A mother-agent is usually the agent or agency that found or discovered you. They basically sign a contract with you, and then sell you to other agencies and markets. They'll make a commission off the commission that the other agencies take.

Portfolio (also called a **book**): A portfolio is a model's résumé in photos—a compilation of photos showing what the model has done in terms of magazines, advertising, and other media. Sometimes it's even just one picture. This is what the model or the model's agent shows to clients.

Showroom: The location where samples of a designer's latest collection are showcased.

Skealthy: Skinny but healthy. (See: **www.urbandictionary.com.**)

■ ■ ■

APPENDIX A

Real Models, Real Meals, Real Modercizing

Supermodel YOU has been full of advice, tips, hints, and stories about how models roll, in order to help you find your supermodel self. But I'll bet you'd love to see some actual model meal plans, read about how real models actually modercize, and even get a few model-tested (and sometimes model-invented) recipes!

That's what this part of the book is all about. I asked lots of models what they eat on a typical day, what kind of physical activity they like to do on a regular basis, and whether they had any meal ideas or recipes they'd like to share. I got hundreds of responses, but I chose the ones I liked the best to share with you here. I know you'll find them inspiring.

You can copy the model menus and meal ideas that look good to you, get motivated by modercizing ideas, and basically get comfortable with your new clique—supermodels! Of course, what you eat and how you move is totally up to you—it's your body and your life. But just like hanging out with friends whose not-so-healthy habits can have a negative impact on your own health habits, reading these pages can be your chance to feel like you're hanging out with friends who have also embraced their supermodel selves. Pretty soon, you'll be inspiring *your* friends to find their supermodel selves, too!

■ ■

JULIE HENDERSON, *Sports Illustrated* supermodel

Breakfast: Breakfast is a hard one for me, as my taste buds take a while to wake up, but I always try to have something. I either go with yogurt with honey, or an egg-white omelette with feta cheese, mushrooms, spinach, and a splash of some type of salsa. I always have my breakfast with a coffee; it really kicks off my day.

Lunch: I almost always have some sort of fish, either sushi or grilled, with rice and veggies.

Dinner: Depending on what my body is craving, I try to feed it what it needs, like steak, chicken, pasta, or even just a light salad. When eating at night, I try to keep the portions small.

Snacks: I love a green juice every couple of days, or sometimes I opt for a handful of mixed nuts or even popcorn.

Modercizing!: I try to stay active most days of the week. I like to alternate running, swimming, yoga, and boxing. Not only does this keep my body interested, but it keeps my mind interested, too.

■ ■

AMANDA FIELDS, international model, runway expert, *Project Runway* model, *America's Next Top Model* guest star, TV host, actress (@TheRunwayQueen on Twitter)

Breakfast: Fruit and coffee.

Lunch: Soup (my favorite soup is tortilla) and salad. I avoid salad dressing because you're literally pouring on calories. Also, I appreciate the flavors of all the ingredients on their own. I do like to add pepper!

Dinner: Chicken and steamed vegetables. I really like cooking at home these days. It's much healthier because you can control how much oil or butter you want in your food.

Snacks: Clif Bars are my very favorite on-set snack. They're also great when I'm going about my day on my castings, auditions, and fittings, so I can stay slim and have energy! I also love to drink Activate, which is water with vitamins in the cap. You twist the cap clockwise to release the vitamins into the water and—voilà—you've got a fresh dose of vitamins that taste great. It's naturally sweetened with a sweetener I love, stevia. Oh, and no calories!

Comments: I definitely eat a wide variety of food! I also allow myself to have a few treats during the week because chocolate makes me so happy. I don't want to deprive myself! Everything in moderation. I'll buy a pack of three cookies instead of a whole box so it doesn't tempt me to go out of control. I definitely stay around 1,800 to 2,000 calories a day.

Modercizing!: My workout regimen is solely The Bar Method. I grew up dancing, doing ballet, tap, and jazz. I really love a class setting with a teacher who encourages you to do that extra curl and get your leg even higher during arabesque! The Bar Method includes interval training, isometrics, dance conditioning, and physical therapy to quickly and safely reshape your entire body! I always say it's like Photoshopping yourself! For more information, go to **www.barmethod.com**.

Supermodel Chefs

I am not the best cook in the world. I'm learning as I go. I would love to learn how to make vegan cookies! I don't consider myself vegan or vegetarian, although I really love to eat that way often!

■ ■

NATALIE PACK, gorgeous fashion model, Miss California USA 2012, pre-medical student at the University of California–Irvine

Breakfast: Five egg whites with two pieces of low-carb toast.

Lunch: Flax tempeh with pesto, and a side salad with walnuts and balsamic vinaigrette.

Dinner: Grilled salmon with lemon and stir-fried veggies.

Snacks: Piece of dark chocolate with 1 cup unsweetened vanilla almond milk; jicama and celery with natural peanut butter; or a handful of unsalted pistachios with 2 teaspoons dried cranberries.

Comments: I typically eat around 1,800 calories a day. I always try to stay below 2,000 calories per day.

Modercizing!: Anything outside of the gym! I love to Rollerblade, bike, and jog outdoors and in the sun. I've recently been taking classes at an indoor trampoline park, and it's an awesome way to exercise and have a blast!

Supermodel Chefs

HEALTHY LOW-CARB RAGU BOLOGNESE

1 medium yellow onion

2 celery stalks

2 medium carrots

2 tablespoons olive oil

1 pound lean ground turkey meat

1 small can tomato paste

1 cup low-sodium chicken stock

Salt and pepper, to taste

1 cup unsweetened soy milk

4 packages Tofu Shirataki noodles

Dice and sauté onion, celery, and carrots in olive oil over medium heat until onions are transparent. Add ground turkey and cook until brown, then add tomato paste and chicken stock, and heat through. Add salt and pepper to taste, then add soy milk to sauce and simmer for up to 1 hour on low heat. If needed, you can add more chicken stock and soy milk. Rinse and drain noodles in a strainer, then microwave in a bowl for 3 minutes. Add sauce, then serve hot.

■ ■

MELISSA ROSE HARO, *Sports Illustrated* Rookie of the Year swimsuit model, 2008–2009

Breakfast: I feel that my mornings are hectic trying to get ready and get out of the house to start my day, so my quick go-to is a protein shake with frozen fruit. On a more relaxed morning, I like to indulge a bit with organic eggs, turkey bacon, and whole-wheat toast. Mmm, so good!

Lunch: Soups and salads are always pretty good and never boring, since there are so many options. I can eat them every day.

Dinner: I eat a lot of lean meats such as turkey and chicken, and just prepare them different ways to keep things interesting.

Snacks: I'm always on the go, so I always have a PowerBar or a bag of nuts and raisins on me. It's so easy, filling, and helps keep my energy up.

Comments: I try to get a lot of B_{12} and vitamin C. I drink approximately 64 ounces of water a day to stay hydrated, and I also love coconut water.

Modercizing!: I don't like to get bored doing the same thing over and over, and I prefer not to realize I'm working out, so I switch off among yoga, swimming, dancing, trying new sports (which I never really get good at, but have a lot of fun doing), walking around the area (I've also made lots of friends this way), and hiking.

Supermodel Chefs

These two recipes are quick, easy, and healthy—and I think they taste great. I make them when I'm preparing for a swimsuit shoot or need to detox.

CABBAGE SOUP

5–8 celery stalks

1 big green cabbage

5 leeks

5 tomatoes

4–5 onions

Splash of white vinegar

Pinch of cloves

Dash of soy sauce

Combine all ingredients and enough water to cover them, and simmer until vegetables are soft. Serve with bread.

MEAN GREEN JUICE

1 bunch of kale

4 stalks of celery

1 cucumber

2 Granny Smith apples

½ lemon

Ginger root (thumb size)

Run all ingredients through a juicer, then sip slowly.

■ ■

EUGENA WASHINGTON, second runner-up on *America's Next Top Model,* represented by Major Model Management New York

Breakfast: Granola cereal with dried cranberries.

Lunch: Protein shake and an apple or a salad.

Dinner: Lots of proteins, like steak or chicken, with broccoli or salad.

Snacks: Apples throughout the day.

Comments: I drink no soda, no coffee, and not really any store-bought juice. I drink two bottles of aloe-vera juice and two bottles of coconut water a day. I try to stay at around 1,500 calories, and I only eat until I'm satisfied but not full. I always carry a snack with me, like an apple, a granola bar, or carrots, so I'm never starving.

Modercizing!: For exercise I take a Zumba class twice a week and yoga three times a week.

Supermodel Chefs

My favorite juice recipes are:

1. A whole pineapple, 2 sweet potatoes, 2 carrots, and 1 orange.

2. A handful of spinach, 2 celery stalks, 1 apple, 1 pear, and a little fresh ginger.

■ ■

BROOKE RITCHIE, model, co-creator of Supermodeled: the site for models by models (**www.supermodeled.com**)

Breakfast: Trader Joe's Blueberry Muesli, almond milk, and plain Greek yogurt and hot green tea or maté blend.

Lunch: Spicy salmon sushi; kale salad; chicken salad with arugula; or a sandwich with lettuce, tomato, and salami.

Dinner: Lean pork tenderloin, roasted veggies, and green beans. Salad with light homemade vinaigrette and steak cooked in butter. Vegetarian pasta without cheese.

Snacks: Raw dried pumpkin seeds, almonds, dried figs, apricots, air-popped popcorn, organic apples, oranges, raspberries, whole-grain crackers and brie cheese. Dark chocolate. Chamomile and green tea. Hot chocolate made with raw cacao.

Comments: I eat small meals often. I try to drink enough tea and water. I rarely have fruit juices, and I love fresh coconut water after a workout. I also try to eat something green (vegetables) with most meals. I really crave salt the most, and if I feel like I need it, I'll have potato chips or dark chocolate as my treat. As long as you're not living on these two things, it's easy to maintain your body and still enjoy what you eat. I also have half a glass of wine or less, twice a week.

Modercizing!: I go to the gym and I hike. If I'm at the gym, I'll warm up my muscles on a bike for 20 minutes, and then run on the treadmill for 20 to 30 minutes. I always stretch afterward to wake up my muscles. I find it relaxing, too. Then I do a mat workout of Pilates and strengthening exercises. I rarely use weights.

Supermodel Chefs

For me, just spending time in the kitchen is a pleasure and a privilege. I'm always adding new vegetables to my repertoire. Educating myself on healthy foods has let me enjoy my food more. Adding foods is always better than taking away foods, and I have found balance in this.

HERBED OMELETTE

2 eggs (with or without yolks)

Splash of milk (any kind you normally use)

Finely chopped herbs

Salt and pepper

Put a pan on medium heat. Lightly beat eggs in a bowl and then add all other ingredients. Put a little butter in the pan and let it melt. Pour in egg mixture. Wait for edges to become firm. Fold omelette over (so it's in half). Then enjoy! The omelette will be firm on the outside and soft in the middle. You can add cheese, but you don't need it.

■ ■

ALEKSANDRA RASTOVIC, superamazing artist and model, represented by VIVA Model Management, Paris

Breakfast: Boiled egg, a cup of nonfat Greek yogurt with a teaspoon of berry jelly for sweetener, old-fashioned oats with a couple of berries on top, and a small cup of coffee with fat-free milk.

Lunch: A salad with everything in it!

Dinner: Grilled or broiled fish and veggies.

Snacks: Fresh juices, particularly from veggies. Currently, as I'm painting in the desert in Southern California and there is plenty of aloe vera around, I've been making a rejuvenating concoction: the juice of a large cucumber, a spoonful of gel from the inside of an aloe vera plant, a small banana, and a teaspoon of brown sugar. The aloe is a bit bitter, but it has incredible benefits in cell rejuvenation. I also drink lattes with soy or nonfat milk. I have chocolate almost every night.

Comments: As a true Mediterranean, I cook everything in olive oil. I also take my eye makeup off with olive oil.

Modercizing!: I get into phases of going to the gym. I'm not a consistent gym person. However, I keep myself active outdoors. When I'm by the beach, I enjoy skateboarding and surfing. Biking is a low-impact workout that I do by the beach or in the city. Right now, I'm hiking in the mountains around my painting studio. Also, I practice jiu-jitsu when I have time. I try to do a set of 15 handstands every day.

Supermodel Chefs

Instead of ranch salad dressing, try Greek yogurt and herbs!

■ ■

EVA SHAW, model, badass DJ (aka "DJ Bambi"; @DJBambi on Twitter)

Breakfast: Vegan protein shake, usually. I'm not a vegan, but this stuff gives me a lot of energy. Sometimes I just eat lunch-type foods. I can eat a sandwich at 9 A.M., no problem!

Lunch: I love big salads. I usually go to New York delis for lunch. I'm a huge soup fan, too. Split pea and turkey chili, *mmm!*

Dinner: I often go out to eat. I love steak, Italian food, Japanese . . . pretty much anything. I like to mix it up. I love a good red wine with dinner.

Snacks: Raw veggies, nuts, hummus, fruit, coffee, Slurpees (LOL), and I have a thing for beef jerky.

Comments: I generally eat pretty healthful foods. My main craving is for red meat. I love burgers and steak. I'm a huge fan of orange soda, too. I rarely eat sweets, but if I do, it's ice cream or M&Ms. I put mustard on almost everything.

Modercizing!: I walk a ton, try to hit the gym, and I dance like no one's watching. I'm a sports fan, too. I love doing anything active.

Supermodel Chefs

I really enjoy cooking, but I don't do it just for myself. Maybe I should start! There's an arugula, fennel, and shaved Parmesan salad I like to make. It's really simple with a nice lemon, olive oil, and mustard dressing. There's nothing like barbecue, though. That's my favorite!

■ ■

DANI LUNDQUIST, international fashion model

Breakfast: I need some protein for breakfast to keep me running smoothly throughout the day, so I will usually make myself an egg with sautéed spinach and garlic and a fresh tomato on the side. Sometimes I'll add a side of lentils for an even more substantial breakfast. I always serve this with whole-wheat toast.

Lunch: I've been really big on making sure I get some raw veggies into my diet lately, so I've been eating a lot of chopped salads. My favorite is a couscous veggie salad. It has equal amounts of couscous (or quinoa), chopped tomatoes, carrots, and cucumber, plus onion and garlic. I always add pumpkin seeds and some chia seeds for some extra omega-3s. I top it with a combination of apple cider vinegar, olive oil, and honey. I like crunchy foods, so I usually have a few water crackers on the side.

Dinner: Being a vegetarian, I try to get really creative in the kitchen to keep things fresh. It's easy and so much fun, and I never miss the meat. Some of my favorites are quinoa-stuffed red peppers, pumpkin soup, veggie stir-fry with brown rice, veggie burgers (which make you feel like you're in heaven), burritos, and enchiladas.

Snacks: Fruit, fruit, and more fruit. Why reach for the bag of chips when you have a super-juicy red apple sitting right in front of you?

Modercizing!: Yoga is my favorite. I'm still trying to really get into it, but I love the way I feel after I have a great class. I'm not that good at going to the gym, but even just getting out and moving is so good. I recently started surfing, and you wouldn't believe the kind of workout that gives you! I've also done a few dance classes, which are great because you're having fun while you're getting exercise. Even finding a friend and going to play tennis or going on a walk and gossiping is always good.

Supermodel Chefs

I live in the kitchen; it's my favorite place in the world. I swear, each apartment I get, the kitchen just keeps getting better and better! I've been doing a ton of homemade recipes lately. I just made my own soy yogurt, which is unbelievably easy. Combine 4 cups of soy milk and ½ cup store-bought organic yogurt. Warm the milk, then whisk in the yogurt. Put in the oven in a covered pan for 8 hours at 100°F and bam!—you have homemade yogurt. It can turn out a bit runny, so you can try adding agar to it, which is a vegetarian gelatin. Even throw in some berries if you'd like. The best part of cooking is that you can do whatever you want! Get creative, have fun, and just enjoy! Food is an experience. Why just throw something in the microwave when you can create your own masterpiece?

■ ■

STEFANIE WOOD, superchef and model, represented by PhotoGenics

Breakfast: Homemade smoothie, oatmeal with maple syrup, or granola with soy milk. I also drink oolong tea.

Lunch: A salad of butter lettuce, avocado, artichoke hearts, tomato, olives (black and green), olive oil, and sea salt.

Dinner: Homemade vegetable soup with quinoa; gluten-free rice pasta with homemade tomato sauce, fresh basil, and fresh mozzarella; or I'll sometimes visit my favorite organic fresh-food restaurant, Puran's, in Los Feliz, California.

Snacks: Seaweed snacks from Trader Joe's, sunflower seed butter, kiwis, apples, pears, pomegranate seeds, carrots, celery, Greek yogurt with cilantro and chives, hummus, rice crackers. Throughout the day, I drink at least two liters of purified water.

Modercizing!: My boyfriend and I hike regularly. Once or twice a week we will do 10- to 13-mile hikes. I don't drive, so I average about three to five miles of walking per day.

Supermodel Chefs

I love cooking and creating my own recipes. I am actually creating a cookbook by myself! Who knows, maybe I'll publish it one day!

ALMOND-BUTTER COOKIES

1 cup unsalted butter

1 cup almond butter

2 cups white sugar

2 eggs

1 teaspoon pure almond extract

2½ cups all-purpose flour

1½ teaspoons baking soda

1 teaspoon baking powder

24 raw almonds

Cream together butter, almond butter, sugar, eggs, and almond extract. Mix together all dry ingredients (except almonds) in a separate bowl and add to wet ingredients gradually while stirring. Chill the dough in the fridge for 15 minutes. Form 1-inch balls of dough and place the balls 1 inch apart from each other on a nonstick baking sheet. Flatten dough balls with a spoon or a fork. Place 1 raw almond on top of each cookie. Bake in a 375°F oven for 9 minutes. Do not overbake.

I love these cookies so much that I make them for my friends. Since one of my friends is vegan, I created a vegan alternative. Simply substitute 1 cup vegan margarine instead of butter, and 4 tablespoons cornstarch instead of eggs.

■ ■

SOPHIA LEE, superstunning Asian American model, represented by Elite Model Management and L.A. Models Runway

Breakfast: Option 1: Oatmeal with golden raisins, mixed nuts (pecan, almond, sunflower seeds, pine nuts, walnuts), and fresh fruit. Option 2: Egg whites with tomato, mushroom, and basil; and wheat bread with flax-seed, nuts, and raisins. Option 3: Fresh smoothies that can be different every time—sometimes with fruit, sometimes with vegetables. I also make my own soy milk.

Lunch: Chinese chicken salad: mixed organic salad with chicken, almonds, oranges, scallions, sesame seeds, carrots, water chestnuts, and ginger sesame dressing. Other options: Chinese noodles with very light chicken broth, and Chinese vegetables lightly cooked with olive oil and sauce. I also like other types of Chinese cooking, mostly vegetable dishes, with fish and white meat. I'm not much of a red-meat person.

Dinner: Salmon very lightly cooked, broccoli on the side. Or Chinese vegetables with tofu and fish-paste balls in light vegetable broth. Another option: dry Chinese noodles with cabbage, mushrooms, chicken, and assorted Chinese condiments. I'm not a big fan of foods that are too heavy on taste and too salty. I'm a very light eater and like food that tastes almost bland (but not tasteless).

Snacks: I eat a lot of fruit, almost enough to make it a meal. I'm always eating fruit. I drink at least eight glasses of water every day. I'm not much of a snacker, and I'm not into chips, fast food, or anything not so healthy. I try to eat all organic if I can. I love tea—I have to drink at least a glass every day to feel good. Chinese people have a habit of drinking tea as a way to flush out toxins and oils after every meal. I drink green tea the most, as it offers many antioxidants.

Modercizing!: I love to do my exercise through shopping and more moderate movements, like lifting up my leg while I'm sitting to get a leg workout, and when shopping, going at a fast pace when I can. I also love dancing and Pilates because they allow me to work out without it being too strenuous!

■ ■

HEATHER CHANTAL JONES, supersweet, wholesome model and *America's Next Top Model* runner-up, 2007

Breakfast: I have either whole-wheat toast with almond butter and honey; fruit; oatmeal; or a cereal high in protein and fiber with almond milk.

Lunch: I usually have a large salad full of all kinds of raw veggies.

Dinner: I usually eat something like quinoa and veggies with fish. Sometimes a pasta. And about once a month, I have red meat for dinner.

Comments: I love dessert! I love dark chocolate, so just about every night I enjoy a few pieces of rich dark chocolate, chocolate-covered almonds, or maybe just a few squares of a bar.

Modercizing!: I love to work out. I think it's very important to get your heart rate up and break a sweat every day. I work out with a personal trainer twice a week lifting light weights and doing resistance training. I love Bikram yoga, and I practice usually three times per week. It makes me feel so strong and healthy! It improves so many things in your life, including your sleep cycle. And speaking of sleep, it's so important! I do my best to get eight hours a night, and often take naps in the afternoon when possible.

Supermodel Chefs

CHIA-SEED PUDDING

This is one healthy dessert I love to make at home. It's delicious, and it's good for you.

Here is the versatile recipe:

½ cup chia seeds

1½ cups almond milk (I love vanilla almond milk)

1 ripe mashed banana

½ tablespoon or less of peanut butter (or any nut butter you'd like)

Mix all ingredients together and let sit for 10 minutes. Stir, then let sit for another 10 minutes. Chill. Makes 2 servings. From here, you can add pretty much anything you'd like to it: berries, nuts, cinnamon, cocoa powder, even chocolate chips. The possibilities are endless, so you'll never get bored!

■ ■

SARA DAVENPORT, my superincredible personal superbooker (my agent) at L.A. Models Runway; chef, personal trainer, holistic health counselor

Breakfast: Green juice and oatmeal with berries.

Lunch: Salad or a veggie wrap.

Dinner: Salad or soup or maybe sushi.

Snacks: Apple and peanut butter or almonds or walnuts.

Comments: I usually only drink water and then coffee. If I'm feeling crazy, I'll have sparkling water! I do know that when I'm stressed, I definitely crave comfort food like pasta and bread. When things are right in my life (work, relationships, spirituality, etc.), then eating healthfully just flows for me.

Modercizing!: I love swimming, surfing, hiking, yoga, spin class, walking and jogging, and lifting weights. I try to work out at least three times per week, but sometimes it's more and sometimes it's less. If my schedule is crazy, I try to at least go for a walk at some point or several points throughout my day just to get my body moving.

Supermodel Chefs

One of my favorite recipes when I want junk food—but don't want to actually eat junk food—is to make sweet-potato nachos. Here's the breakdown:

Take a big sweet potato and slice it into thin slices, like ¼ inches. Put them on a baking sheet. Use parchment paper on the baking sheet to keep them from sticking; that way, you don't have to use any oil. Sprinkle smoked paprika on them, and bake at 350°F to 400°F for 30 minutes. Flip them halfway through to make sure they cook evenly and all the way through. Arrange the slices on a plate and top with your favorite nacho goodies; I usually use black beans, fresh salsa, avocados, and cilantro. Superdelicious, nutritious, filling, and it feels like such a treat!

■ ■

JENNIFER McMANIS, mommy first, model second

Breakfast: On a typical day, I have a venti iced caramel macchiato with extra caramel sauce. If I'm feeling fat or bloated, then I'll get a venti iced skinny vanilla latte. Usually I'll eat a little cereal with fresh berries or yogurt with honey, or have a muffin. But always a venti coffee in the morning. Always. Every Sunday I have eggs Benedict and home fries or potatoes, with a mimosa (if I had a chill night) for brunch. If it was a rage night, I go with ginger ale—best thing for a hangover. I've been known to be one of the first people in line at In-N-Out at 10:30 A.M. when they open. I always order a cheeseburger with extra cheese, 7UP, and fries. I never end up finishing the fries, though.

Lunch: I usually skip lunch or eat extremely small portions. If I'm on set, I must eat! I usually get a salad, dressing on the side, or it gets soggy. Getting dressing on the side is smart because then you can take the leftovers home. I hate to waste food.

Dinner: I usually eat a large dinner. If I'm with my kids, it's early, like 6 to 7 P.M. If I'm out to eat, it's usually 8 to 8:30 P.M. I feel old, but eating after 10 P.M. is just not for me anymore, unless I'm on vacation.

Snacks: I don't really do a lot of snacking—hardly ever. I don't get very hungry during the day, until about noon to 2 P.M. I'm the best at dips, though: crab dip, seven-layer dip, avocado, salsa—all of them. That's the only time I snack. But it's usually on the weekend. Or at a cookout. I drink smart water for electrolytes.

Comments: I love to grill out—burgers, steaks, hot dogs. I like teas and try to avoid soda during the day. I don't eat corn or red cabbage. I'm a decent cook, but don't like to skimp on taste, so I don't cut a ton of calories. Plus, my kids would kill me if I tried to feed them nothing but Lean Cuisine meals. Last night we ordered thin-crust cheese pizza; I had three slices. My boyfriend, my kids, and I always partake in taco Tuesday, and I make it a little more healthy by using turkey instead of ground beef. It tastes better, and it's easier to cook. I also like to bake. Cupcakes are my specialty and so easy. Kids love them, and I always make variations so everyone is happy. I attempt chocolate-chip cookies a couple times a year. I do have one secret: every night, I mix whole organic psyllium husk in cranberry or orange juice. It helps your digestive tract. You can find it at places like Henry's, Sprouts, Whole Foods, etc. I have no idea how many calories I take in on a typical day. Sometimes those numbers are probably off the charts, but I try to balance my unhealthy days with my more food-productive days. A splurge day is always good. Mine is usually the entire weekend!

Modercizing!: I don't work out because I'm already so busy. If I'm not running after a four- or seven-year-old or toting them to and from school, I'm running around the city to castings or doing direct bookings out of state.

■ ■

TRINETTE FAINT, former model, writer, entrepreneur
(**www.trinettefaintproductions.com** and **www.lovehue.com**)

Breakfast: Boiled egg, toast, and smoothie.

Lunch: Usually chicken with veggies.

Dinner: Fish with salad and veggies or beets with arugula.

Snacks: Raw nuts, hummus, and Sesame Blues chips.

Comments: I don't limit myself with food, but I do everything in moderation and make small changes that make a big difference, like eating whole-wheat products, drinking lots of water, eating organics, not eating too much meat, and eating minimal desserts. Fortunately, I don't have a sweet tooth, but rather a healthy appetite!

Modercizing!: I go to the gym four times a week, where I do Pilates, yoga, strength training (weights), and spinning. I also walk a lot every day.

Supermodel Chefs

I love chicken parmesan, and I alter it by sautéing the chicken in olive oil and using whole-wheat pasta. If I'm using flour as a batter for the chicken and not bread crumbs, I use whole-wheat flour. I never measure anything, but this is the general idea. You can also put the chicken in the oven if you're using bread crumbs.

CHICKEN PARMESAN WITH WHOLE-WHEAT PASTA

1 chicken breast

1 egg, beaten

¼ cup bread crumbs without high-fructose corn syrup, or whole-wheat flour

1 teaspoon olive oil

2 garlic cloves, chopped

2–3 tomatoes, chopped

½ cup whole-wheat pasta

1–2 ounces fresh mozzarella, sliced

Salt and pepper, to taste

Season chicken with salt and pepper, soak in egg, roll in bread crumbs or flour, and place in baking dish with olive oil. Bake in the oven 15–20 minutes or until chicken is cooked through.

Sauté garlic cloves and a generous amount of chopped tomatoes. Set aside a small portion of cooked mixture. Add cooked whole-wheat pasta to pan with remaining garlic and tomatoes, and stir.

After both pasta and chicken are done, place chicken on top of pasta, and top with fresh mozzarella. Top with the additional garlic and tomatoes. Place in oven for about 5 minutes, or until cheese is melted. Enjoy!

■ ■

BRYNN JONES, model, represented by PhotoGenics

Breakfast: Coffee, one egg, English muffin, or something fancy made by my boyfriend.

Lunch: Veggie sandwich or salad.

Dinner: Something usually very cheesy and Italian with a salad, bread, and a cocktail.

Snack: Soy yogurt with granola; a protein bar; something chocolate.

Comments: I never eat meat because I'm a vegetarian. Roughly three days a week, I consume two to five cocktails (*shhh . . . !*).

Modercizing!: I love to hike from time to time, more to clear my mind than for exercise, but subconsciously I credit myself for the cardio that my mind-clearing hike provides.

Supermodel Chefs

Here are two great beverage recipes, courtesy of Brenda Vongova, supermodel trainer and founder of the Vongova Body Lift method. Each makes 1 serving.

GINGER TONIC

1 cup mineral water (without artificially added CO_2; such as Gerolsteiner)

1 teaspoon ginger extract

2–4 drops liquid stevia

NONALCOHOLIC WINE

1 cup grape kombucha

1 teaspoon resveratrol extract (the heart-healthy component of red wine)

■ ■ ■

APPENDIX B

Five Keys Resources

Modeling-industry websites:

Daily Front Row: **www.fashionweekdaily.com**

Modelinia: **www.modelinia.com**

Models.com: **www.models.com**

Style.com: **www.style.com**

TheOnes2Watch.com: **theones2watch.com**

Women's Wear Daily: **www.wwd.com**

Supermodel role-model websites:

Tyra Banks: **www.tyrabanks.com**

Gisele Bündchen: **www.giselebundchen.com**

Cindy Crawford: **www.cindy.com**

Kathy Ireland: **www.kathyireland.com**

Miranda Kerr: **www.mirandakerr.net**

Heidi Klum: **www.heidiklum.aol.com**

Christy Turlington: **www.everymothercounts.org**

Healthy-living websites:

The Beauté Guru: **www.beauteguru.com/about**

The Beauty Bean: **www.thebeautybean.com**

The Daily Love: **www.thedailylove.com**

DeepakChopra.com: **www.deepakchopra.com**

Fitness magazine: **www.fitnessmagazine.com**

Fit Tip Daily: **www.fittipdaily.com**

FLO Living: **www.floliving.com**

Heal Your Life: **www.healyourlife.com**

Her Future: **www.herfuture.com**

MindBodyGreen: **www.mindbodygreen.com**

The Model Alliance: **www.modelalliance.org**

Oprah.com: **www.oprah.com**

Owning Pink: **www.owningpink.com**

Positively Positive: **www.positivelypositive.com**

Proud2Bme: **www.proud2bme.org**

Self magazine: **www.self.com**

The Sleep Doctor: **www.thesleepdoctor.com**

Supermodeled: **www.supermodeled.com**

Women's Health magazine: **www.womenshealthmag.com**

Books I love:

Beauty Sleep: Look Younger, Lose Weight, and Feel Great Through Better Sleep, by Michael Breus, Ph.D.

The Biology of Belief: Unleashing the Power of Consciousness, Matter & Miracles, by Bruce Lipton, Ph.D.

Change Your Brain, Change Your Body: Use Your Brain to Get and Keep the Body You Have Always Wanted, by Daniel G. Amen, M.D.

Constant Cravings: What Your Food Cravings Mean and How to Overcome Them, by Doreen Virtue

A Course in Weight Loss: 21 Spiritual Lessons for Surrendering Your Weight Forever, by Marianne Williamson

The Energy Balance Diet: Lose Weight, Control Your Cravings, and Even Out Your Energy, by Joshua Rosenthal and Tom Monte

Fit for Life, Not Fat for Life, by Harvey Diamond

The 4-Hour Body: An Uncommon Guide to Rapid Fat-Loss, Incredible Sex, and Becoming Superhuman, by Timothy Ferriss

Heal Your Body: The Mental Causes for Physical Illness and the Metaphysical Way to Overcome Them, by Louise L. Hay

The Intention Experiment: Using Your Thoughts to Change Your Life and the World, by Lynne McTaggart

Molecules of Emotion: The Science Behind Mind-Body Medicine, by Candace B. Pert, Ph.D.

Perfect Health: The Complete Mind/Body Guide, by Deepak Chopra, M.D.

Skinny Bitch: A No-Nonsense, Tough-Love Guide for Savvy Girls Who Want to Stop Eating Crap and Start Looking Fabulous, by Kim Barnouin and Rory Freedman

Women, Food, and God: An Unexpected Path to Almost Everything, by Geneen Roth

YOU on a Diet: The Owner's Manual for Waist Management, by Michael F. Roizen, M.D., and Mehmet C. Oz, M.D. (aka "Dr. Oz")

My favorite calorie-counter/fitness-tracking apps:

Calorie Counter by FatSecret

Calorie Counter by MyNetDiary

DailyBurn

Eat This Not That! The Game

Lose It!

MyFitnessPal

Noom Weight Loss Coach

Beauty-sleep accessories:

Earplugs: Mack's (**www.macksearplugs.com**) are the model-approved ones. Available at drugstores.

Eye mask: Bucky's (**www.bucky.com**) or Aroma Home (**http:// us.aromahome.com**), or any eye mask you find comfortable.

Melatonin: Melatonin is a natural sleep aid also known to help with jet lag. Many models use melatonin for sleep and travel. Available at drugstores.

More cool stuff:

Elle magazine: **www.elle.com**

Hay House (they publish the best books for getting your life into balance!): **www.hayhouse.com**

FabSugar (style news): **www.fabsugar.com**

TellMeLater app (set modeltude reminders—your posture, positive affirmations, etc.): download from iTunes

Vogue magazine: **www.vogue.com**

■ ■ ■

APPENDIX C

Eating Disorders Information and Resources

I hope you never have to grapple with an eating disorder, but if you do, please consult these excellent resources for help.

Academy for Eating Disorders (AED) is a multidisciplinary professional organization that focuses on anorexia nervosa, bulimia nervosa, binge eating disorder, and related disorders. They sponsor a newsletter and a conference. Find them on the web at: **www.aedweb.org**.

Binge Eating Disorder Association (BEDA) is the national organization focusing on increased prevention, diagnosis, and treatment for binge eating disorder. Find them on the web at: **www.bedaonline.com**.

Eating Disorder Hope is a website at **www.eatingdisorderhope.com** that promotes ending disordered eating behavior, embracing life, and pursuing recovery.

Eating Disorders Anonymous provides information about local support-group meetings. Find them on the web at: **www.eatingdisorders anonymous.org**.

National Eating Disorders Association (NEDA) is a nonprofit organization dedicated to supporting individuals and families affected by eating disorders. NEDA has been so supportive of *Supermodel YOU* and my mission, and they are an amazing organization that does so much good work. Find them on the web at **www.nationaleatingdisorders.org**, or call the toll-free National Information and Referral Helpline at (800) 931-2237.

Irene Rubaum-Keller, LMFT, is a psychotherapist with more than 20 years of experience in treating people with eating disorders. There is extensive information on her website about all forms of eating disorders. She is the author of the book *Foodaholic* and is also on staff at UCLA. She is available in person at her office in Los Angeles, and by phone for those outside the L.A. area. Find her on the web at **www.eatingdisorder therapist.com**, or call (310) 474-2208.

■ ■ ■

ACKNOWLEDGMENTS

Writing these Acknowledgments has been even harder for me than writing this book, but worth the effort because I believe acknowledging the people who have contributed to it, inspired it, and kept me believing in myself and in this project even when it felt like it was never going to happen deserve my most sincere thanks. So while I can't possibly thank everyone (that would be an entire book in itself), first and foremost, I want to thank *you*, my readers! Every day, we are bombarded with a bazillion different things begging for our attention, but right now, in this moment, I have yours, and I appreciate that more than you can imagine. I also want to tell you something very important: If you believe in something and are passionate about it, *never* give up on it. You've helped me do that in my life, and I hope this book helps you do the same.

I must also thank some others by name. This book never would have been possible if I hadn't been given the opportunity to model in the first place, so to Nicole Bordeaux at PhotoGenics, who "found" me, and together with your amazing team of believers at PhotoGenics, "made" me, thank you! It's funny to say I was found, but in many ways, yes, I was lost before you. To the rest of my PhotoGenics family (Melanie, Nicci, Rick, Emily, Marcus, Justin, Jane, and Phira), your continued belief in me as a model and now as an author/spokesperson is something I truly cherish. Phira Luon, you are not only an amazing agent, you are an incredible person, and any model should be honored to call you their agent.

To Crista Klayman at L.A. Models Runway, you are my lifesaver and my angel. You sparkled fairy dust on me. A girl never forgets where she got her wings! To the rest of my beloved runway agents and team at L.A. Models (Lauren, Daniel, Domino, Huey, Anahid, Sarah, Kimberly, Rita, Paul, and Heinz), I appreciate all of you!

Melissa Ghirimoldi at Muse NY, I can't say enough about what your loyalty means to me. I hold you in such high regard and am honored to have you represent me! To the rest of my rocking team of agents in New York at Muse (Conor, Ed, Juana, Emily, Jeanna, Erin, Becca, Julie, Lanny, Jessica, Ariana, Sidra, and Shakira), thank you for keeping me on the board even when I'm not in New York and for always keeping faith in me and this book.

One model, so many agents (and I've only mentioned the ones in the U.S. in the fashion industry)! I can't not mention Wendy Levene Goldberg, Jon Tutulo, Marco Amato, and Guillaume Terrasson, who first represented me worldwide and who truly believed in that insecure, clueless, small-town girl. To my other notable bookers, Sara Davenport, Karina Dial, Francis Enriquez, and Tuomas Ahonen, all of you have allowed me to get to where I am today, and I remain so grateful to have had your support. If you ever represented me, pushed me to a client, booked me a job, or believed in me— even if it was purely based on my "alien look"—from the bottom of heart, I thank you!

To all the beautiful and amazing models and supermodels all over the world I have had the opportunity to know, work with, live with, travel with, laugh with, and cry and complain with, thank you for inspiring this book! Some of you are now among my greatest friends. Thank you for your contribution both directly and indirectly.

To the sometimes crazy but also amazing fashion industry and all my wonderful and loyal clients, thank you for letting me represent your brands. I am continually honored to shoot for you, walk for you, and work for you. To each and every person involved in the casting aspects who has booked me over and over again, I owe you endless appreciation and always strive to live up to the image, look, and feel of the job at hand.

To my SuperBoys: Rob Corbett, you of all people are closest to this project, and your advice, help, comments, and everything you've done have been my fuel to continue pursuing this when I was often discouraged. I can't thank you enough. I truly love you! David Chacon, thank you for pointing out that health, fitness, and helping others was my true passion in life. Ryan Daly, you took the first initiative by putting your name out there for me before anyone else. I will always remember that! Matt Heagy, you know firsthand how dedicated and married I was and am to this book. Thank you for being there for me and believing in me. Jeremy Brown, at Throne Publishing, you've been my unofficial publishing advisor. Thanks for always guiding me in the right direction. Stuart Johnson at *Success* magazine, I met you only days before delivering this manuscript, yet your influence on me will be instrumental in this book's and my personal success going forward. Marcellas Reynolds, I treasure your continued support and affection. John Tew, my Beauté Guru and dear friend, you are a gift. To my other guru, Guru Mirumi, Ph.D., without a healthy mind and body, accomplishing anything would have been impossible. I am grateful you came into my life when you did. Cameron Silver, *j'adore*. Period. Rob Meadows, Jason Bleick, Christopher Phillips, Chad Keller, Todd Sandler, Brad Bode, Paul Weinberg, and Rob Hollister, you have been there for me personally and in regards to this book in more ways than I can express. You will always be an integral and important part of my life. I love you guys!

To my SuperGirls: I am inspired by every woman and girl I meet in my life! To all the gorgeous girls in my life, I love you: Ginger Lewis, you are my soul sister. To my lifelong girlfriends, Kristine Naumova Ureña, Renie Toyama, Michelle Meekins, Mandy Nicole Whitley, Christy Pecyna, Rebecca Deanna, Helene Smith, Amber Lane, Cristine Byrns, Patricia Chacon, and Shay Londre Weinberg, all of you have been in my life a long time and always will be regardless of the distance and time that divides us. Courtney Marinovich, we just met, but I have a feeling we'll be friends a long time. To all the other influential and supportive women who have helped specifically in regards to this book and who have aided my dreams, thank you for your support, friendship, and inspiration: Ashley

Conrad, Janice Heagy, Trinette Faint, Melanie De Jesus, Agapi Stassinopoulos, Janine Francolini, Brenda Vongova, Terri Cole, Michelle Phillips, and all the models and people who are quoted in this book.

Melissa Rodwell, beautiful people take beautiful pictures. Thank you for shooting this book cover and for always supporting my career. To the style icon Ms. Kate Lanphear, you're amazing. Thank you for your book-cover tips! And to Lynn Grefe at the National Eating Disorder Association, thank you for helping me guide girls in a better direction and for your endless advice and counsel. I promise to honor your request and continue to support what you do at NEDA.

Health and fitness has always been a huge passion of mine ever since *Sweating to the Oldies* in diapers with my mom and Richard Simmons. My health-and-fitness community is a huge part of my life and a major inspiration to me. Keith Levin, you introduced me to yoga. I am so grateful for you and our yoga group—I love all of you like family! Jennifer Pastiloff, your unique teaching styles, from manifestation yoga to Karaoke Yoga, have inspired me and so many to join your tribe. Philip Kessel, aka PK, you inspire so many of us, and we all remain loyal to you, your music, and the energy and love you pour into every class! Aimée Donahue, your knowledge about the body and mind fascinates me. And to my amazing friend and instructor April Bernardi, you introduced to me a whole new way of using my mind, my energy, my spirit, and my body. Many of my breakthroughs began after taking your first class. We are forever connected, and the inspiration you've unknowingly contributed to my life is extraordinary. I can only hope to do the same for you. I love you, girl!

To Hay House, my publisher, OMG! You were and are my dream publisher. I believe wholeheartedly in what you do and what you stand for. Louise Hay, you have built an empire out of changing people's lives. For me to be a part of what you're doing is an incredible honor. Reid Tracy, thank you so much for this amazing opportunity that you have given me. I can only aspire to live up to the Hay House legacy as a person and author! To Alex Freemon and Shannon Littrell, who first saw my proposal and ended up editing this book, thank you, thank you, thank you! Gail Gonzales,

Erin Dupree, Nancy Levin, Stacey Smith, Cheryl Richardson, and the whole ridiculously awesome and amazing team of people and authors at Hay House, I have endless appreciation for all of you and truly admire what you do.

Eve Adamson, my glorious co-writer. I could never have written this book without you. You were my dream writer! Yay! You are truly gifted, and your contribution to this book was invaluable.

To all the amazing people who have inspired me through their work, have written endorsements, or who have given me support and guidance, I am truly honored and grateful: Dr. Darren R. Weissman; Alain Morin, Ph.D.; Dr. Kristen G. Hairston; Linda Sivertsen; Irene Rubaum-Keller, LMFT; Daniel Stone, D.C.; Greg James; Amanda Luttrell Garrigus; Brent Huff; Eric Handler; Ryan J. Blair; Lauren Galit; Greg Alterman; Derek Blasberg; Mastin Kipp; Michael J. Chase; Steven Bell; Andrew Macpherson; Melissa Lamming; Roxy; Tony Jeary; Alonna Travin; Kristin Barone; Kenn Henman; Jonathon R. Stein; Shannon Davidson; Dr. Sanusi Uma; and everyone who has influenced me and this book (just insert your name here if I forgot you: _____), I offer you my super-appreciation and endless respect and love.

To everyone else, on Twitter, on Facebook, and everywhere else where we've interacted, *you* are my daily inspiration! I love you. I appreciate you. And I hope this book helps you find *your* beautiful inner supermodel self.

Lastly, to my family, who will read this book someday and probably not like everything written in regard to our past, know that I am telling my story from my perspective. You also have yours. No matter what, I love our story. It has made us who we are today and who we will become tomorrow. I am very proud of where we all stand. I love you and have nothing but endless, compassionate, and unconditional love and respect for all of you. Each and every one of you means the world to me, but nieces and nephews are the biggest joy in my heart! Someday, we will be a family again and realize that our trials and tribulations were our greatest blessings in disguise.

— Sarah DeAnna

■ ■

I never imagined I'd be writing about models, but when Sarah DeAnna contacted me asking for some help with her manuscript, I couldn't resist her charm, unique voice, irresistible idea, and obvious inner beauty. Thanks, Sarah, for a wonderful experience! I must also thank my assistant, Hannah Rounds, for diligent and enthusiastic proofreading, and the whole Hay House team for their support, enthusiasm, and crackerjack editing job. Everything about this book has been super.

— Eve Adamson

■ ■ ■

ABOUT THE AUTHORS

Overcoming childhood poverty and personal tragedy, **Sarah DeAnna** graduated high school with honors, then put herself through college, earning a degree in international business marketing. After college, Sarah was "discovered" and went on to become a successful international high-fashion model who has appeared in some of the biggest and most influential fashion magazines worldwide, including *Vogue, Elle, Marie Claire, Amica, L'Officiel,* and *Riviera.* She has done runway shows and other events for renowned designers, including Dolce & Gabbana, Versace, and Stella McCartney, among others. She has also appeared as a model on various TV segments for stations and shows such as TLC, Bravo, MTV, E!, *Hollywood Insider,* and *Good Morning America.* Sarah is represented by several agencies worldwide.

One of the reasons Sarah is so successful in the modeling industry is because of her commitment to a healthy, balanced lifestyle. She is fascinated by nutrition and wellness, and is also committed to compassionate living and spreading the message to women and young girls that beauty radiates from within—and that self-love, confidence, and a commitment to health are what make every woman just as gorgeous as any supermodel.

Website: **www.sarahdeanna.com**

■ ■

Eve Adamson is a four-time *New York Times* best-selling author and multiple award-winning freelance writer who has written or co-written more than 50 books, including all four of TV star Bethenny Frankel's bestsellers: *Naturally Thin, The Skinnygirl Dish, A Place of Yes,* and the novel *Skinnydipping.* Eve specializes in collaborating with celebrities and experts on books about dieting, holistic health, cooking, personal development, fitness, business, and animals. She also writes memoirs and novels, and has penned hundreds of magazine articles over the course of her 17-year career. Eve and Sarah share passions for natural foods, health, yoga, beauty secrets, compassionate living, and veganism.

Website: **www.eveadamson.com**

■ ■ ■

We hope you enjoyed this Hay House book. If you'd like to
receive our online catalog featuring additional information on
Hay House books and products, or if you'd like to find out
more about the Hay Foundation, please contact:

Hay House, Inc., P.O. Box 5100, Carlsbad, CA 92018-5100
(760) 431-7695 or (800) 654-5126
(760) 431-6948 (fax) or (800) 650-5115 (fax)
www.hayhouse.com® • **www.hayfoundation.org**

■ ■ ■

Published and distributed in Australia by:
Hay House Australia Pty. Ltd., 18/36 Ralph St., Alexandria NSW 2015 •
Phone: 612-9669-4299 • *Fax:* 612-9669-4144 • www.hayhouse.com.au

Published and distributed in the United Kingdom by:
Hay House UK, Ltd., Astley House, 33 Notting Hill Gate, London W11 3JQ •
Phone: 44-20-3675-2450 • *Fax:* 44-20-3675-2451 • www.hayhouse.co.uk

Published and distributed in the Republic of South Africa by:
Hay House SA (Pty), Ltd., P.O. Box 990, Witkoppen 2068 •
Phone/Fax: 27-11-467-8904 • www.hayhouse.co.za

Published in India by: Hay House Publishers India, Muskaan Complex,
Plot No. 3, B-2, Vasant Kunj, New Delhi 110 070 • *Phone:* 91-11-4176-1620 •
Fax: 91-11-4176-1630 • www.hayhouse.co.in

Distributed in Canada by:
Raincoast, 9050 Shaughnessy St., Vancouver, B.C. V6P 6E5 •
Phone: (604) 323-7100 • *Fax:* (604) 323-2600 • www.raincoast.com

■ ■ ■

Take Your Soul on a Vacation

Visit **www.HealYourLife.com®** to regroup, recharge, and reconnect
with your own magnificence. Featuring blogs, mind-body-spirit news,
and life-changing wisdom from Louise Hay and friends.

Visit **www.HealYourLife.com** today!